BEAT
CANCER
DAILY

Published in the United States by: Hay House LLC: www.hayhouse.com® • **Published in Australia by:** Hay House Australia Publishing Pty Ltd: www.hayhouse.com.au • **Published in the United Kingdom by:** Hay House UK Ltd: www.hayhouse.co.uk • **Published in India by:** Hay House Publishers (India) Pvt Ltd: www.hayhouse.co.in

Scripture used by permission of:
ESV® Bible (The Holy Bible, English Standard Version®)
Copyright © 2001 by Crossway, a publishing ministry of Good News Publishers. Used by permission. All rights reserved.

Holman Christian Standard Bible® (HCSB)
Used by permission HCSB © 1999, 2000, 2002, 2003, 2009 by Holman Bible Publishers. Holman Christian Standard Bible®, Holman CSB®, and HCSB® are federally registered trademarks of Holman Bible Publishers.

New American Standard Bible® (NASB)
Copyright © 1960, 1962, 1963, 1968, 1971, 1972, 1973, 1975, 1977, 1995 by The Lockman Foundation. Used by permission. www.Lockman.org.

New International Version (NIV)
Holy Bible, New International Version®, NIV® Copyright ©1973, 1978, 1984, 2011 by Biblica, Inc.™ Used by permission of Zondervan. All rights reserved worldwide. www.zondervan.com. The "NIV" and "New International Version" are trademarks registered in the United States Patent and Trademark Office by Biblica, Inc.™

New King James Version (NKJV)
Scripture taken from the New King James Version®. Copyright © 1982 by Thomas Nelson. Used by permission. All rights reserved.

New Living Translation (NLT)
Holy Bible, New Living Translation, copyright © 1996, 2004, 2015 by Tyndale House Foundation. Used by permission of Tyndale House Publishers, Inc., Carol Stream, Illinois 60188. All rights reserved.

Cover design: Tricia Breidenthal • *Interior design:* Nick C. Welch

Library of Congress has cataloged the earlier edition as follows:

Names: Wark, Chris, author.
Title: Beat cancer daily : 365 days of inspiration, encouragement, and
    action steps to survive and thrive / Chris Wark.
Description: 1st edition. | Carlsbad : Hay House, Inc., 2020. |
Identifiers: LCCN 2020035854 | ISBN 9781401961947 (hardback) | ISBN
    9781401961954 (ebook)
Subjects: LCSH: Cancer--Popular works. | Cancer--Patients--Popular works. |
    Self-care, Health--Popular works.
Classification: LCC RC263 .W34 2020 | DDC 616.99/4--dc23
LC record available at https://lccn.loc.gov/2020035854

Tradepaper ISBN: 978-1-4019-6343-9
E-book ISBN: 978-1-4019-6195-4

11 10 9 8 7 6 5 4 3 2
1st edition, October 2020
2nd edition, September 2022

Printed in the United States of America

This product uses responsibly sourced papers and/or recycled materials. For more information, see www.hayhouse.com.

SUSTAINABLE FORESTRY INITIATIVE

Certified Chain of Custody
Promoting Sustainable Forestry
www.forests.org
SFI-01268

SFI label applies to the text stock

BEAT CANCER DAILY

365 DAYS OF INSPIRATION, ENCOURAGEMENT, AND ACTION STEPS TO SURVIVE AND THRIVE

CHRIS WARK

HAY HOUSE LLC
Carlsbad, California • New York City
London • Sydney • New Delhi

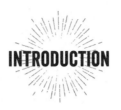

INTRODUCTION

Welcome to *Beat Cancer Daily*! If you don't know my story, I was diagnosed with stage IIIc colon cancer at 26 years old. After surgery I opted out of chemotherapy and embarked on a holistic healing adventure, which is detailed in my first book, *Chris Beat Cancer: A Comprehensive Plan for Healing Naturally*. This journey changed my life and taught me invaluable lessons about life and death, faith and fear, self-care and survival. Over the last 16 years I've had the privilege of studying and learning from many other doctors, experts, and survivors.

I also created a video course for cancer patients, their loved ones, and those interested in prevention, called the *SQUARE ONE Cancer Coaching Program*.

I wrote *Beat Cancer Daily* to give you daily inspiration, encouragement, and action steps to help you survive and thrive. Every day is an opportunity for change and growth—mentally, physically, emotionally, and spiritually. The intention of this book is to help you work through the process of radical life change. To help you make your life simpler yet richer. To help you take control of your health, to help you face your fears, to help you fan the flames of faith, to help you let go of the past, and to help you embrace the present and be hopeful about the future.

There are recurring themes throughout this book because sometimes you need to hear the same piece of advice two or three or ten times before it sinks in. This book will challenge you in the best way possible. It will challenge you to examine your life from every angle, to think differently, to push through resistance, and to take massive action. I didn't just write this book to help you; I wrote it to help me too. Even though I don't have cancer anymore, I need this encouragement, advice, inspiration, and motivation every single day, just like you.

My prayer for you is that you prosper in good health even as your soul prospers.

And that you *beat cancer daily*!

—**Chris**

Join my email newsletter:
www.chrisbeatcancer.com

Join my social media communities:

 www.facebook.com/chrisbeatcancer

 www.youtube.com/chrisbeatcancer

 www.instagram.com/chrisbeatcancer

Learn more about the *SQUARE ONE Cancer Coaching Program*: **www.chrisbeatcancer.com/coaching**

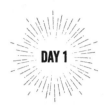

DAY 1

This is the day which the Lord has made;
Let us rejoice and be glad in it.

—Psalm 118:24 (NASB)

Most days, this is the first verse I think of as soon as I wake up. It reminds me that God is the Creator of life, the Creator of the universe, and the Creator of today.

Cancer taught me how precious life is and to thank God for every new day of life.

God created today, and you can trust Him to get you through it.

Happiness is a choice. You can choose to be glad.

Rejoice means to be joyful. You can choose to be joyful.

Gratitude is also a choice. You can choose to be thankful for another day of life and for every single thing you have.

Stir up your happiness by doing things that happy people do. Smile, laugh, sing, dance! This is the day the Lord has made. Rejoice and be glad in it!

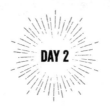

DAY 2

Welcome to the University of Cancer Survival, aka Cancer College. You are now enrolled as a full-time student.

Your self-directed course curriculum should be tailored to provide you with expertise in your cancer type, the benefits and risks of treatments, anti-cancer nutrition, exercise, detoxification, mindset, stress reduction, faith, fear, and forgiveness.

The quality of the education you receive will be directly proportional to your enthusiasm to learn, your willingness to set aside your preconceived notions, your openness to consider new information and ideas, and your commitment to put your newly acquired knowledge to use and to change every aspect of your life.

There's a lot to learn and a lot to do, but don't let yourself feel overwhelmed. You are smart and capable. You can do this!

Be organized, diligent, patient, and persistent. Keep searching and keep learning. And trust that the answers, help, information, and resources you need will come to you at the perfect time.

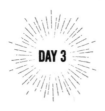

DAY 3

CANCER IS A DIVINE TAP ON THE SHOULDER

In 2003 my body was trying to get my attention. And the message was, "Hey, the way you are living is killing you!" I realized that I alone was responsible for my life and health, no one else. And if I had inadvertently contributed to my illness, then I could also deliberately contribute to my wellness. This revelation, free of blame or shame, snapped me out of complacency and victimhood and empowered me to take massive action to radically change my life. If you have cancer, your body is trying to tell you the same thing. Your survival is not a coin toss. It's not a casino bet. You have the power to affect your future, to stack the odds in your favor with your daily choices. Now is the time to make deliberate life- and health-promoting choices each day. Your choices matter!

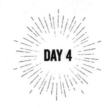

DO YOU?

There's a big difference between not dying and truly living. If you've been diagnosed with cancer or a terminal illness, you may initially be focused on not dying, but the most powerful question you can ask yourself is this:

Do I want to live?

If your answer is yes, my next question for you is "Why?" Why do you want to live? If you aren't sure, take a few minutes to think about what you have to live for. Your reasons to live might be people in your life who need you, people you want to love and serve. Your reason might be a purpose, a calling, a mission you haven't accomplished, a dream you haven't fulfilled, or it might be all of the above. Now is the time to get really clear on this.

Today's Challenge: *Make a list of your reasons to live and put this list in places where you will see it every day. Tack the list on the wall. Write it on your bathroom mirror. Make it the background on your computer screen. Make it the lock screen on your phone. Keeping your reasons to live in front of you and on your mind throughout the day will help keep you focused and determined in moments of weakness and doubt.*

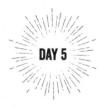

DAY 5

TRUST IN THE LORD

Trust in the Lord with all your heart. And do not lean on your own understanding. In all your ways acknowledge Him, And He will make your paths straight.

—PROVERBS 3:5–6 (NASB)

This is a simple command with a promise attached to it.

Trust that God has a plan, even when you don't understand.

Submit to Him and honor Him in everything you do.

And He will make your path straight.

A straight path is what you want. It's the shortest and fastest way to get to where you want to go. No sidetracks, detours, or wild goose chases that waste your time, effort, energy, and money.

Lord, I trust you with my life, my health, my family, and my future. I submit to you and commit to honor you in what I say and do today. Thank you for directing my path and making it straight. Amen.

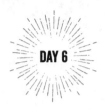

DAY 6

THE BEAT CANCER MINDSET

In the 17 years since my cancer diagnosis, I've read about, met, and interviewed many people who have healed all types and stages of cancer. And they all shared the same belief.

They believed they could get well.[1]

This is the single most important factor—the linchpin in every successful healing story. And they had what I call the Beat Cancer Mindset, which has five components:

Accept total responsibility for your health.
You are the driver of your healing journey.

Be willing to do whatever it takes.
This means changing everything.

Take massive action.
Massive action produces massive results.

Make plans for the future.
Plan to survive and thrive. See yourself well.

Enjoy your life and the process.
Embrace your healing adventure with joy!

---

1 Learn from holistic survivors at www.chrisbeatcancer.com/survivors.

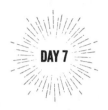

POINT YOUR SHIP TOWARD HEALTHY ISLAND

Improving or restoring your health is a journey.

Healthy Island is the destination.

And it takes time to get there.

You are the captain of your ship. You are at the wheel. You control the rudder.

Some days are easy—the sun is shining, the wind is at your back, and it's smooth sailing.

Other days it's hard to tell if you're getting anywhere.

And some days the wind and the rain, the choppy waves, and the storms of life are rough. They beat you up. And you have to fight to maintain your direction. And sometimes you still get knocked off course. But that's okay.

As the African proverb says, "Smooth seas do not make skillful sailors."

Remember: setbacks and mistakes only defeat you if you quit. When you get knocked off course—it will happen—just point your ship back toward Healthy Island and keep sailing.

One day at a time. One wave at a time.

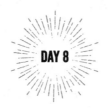

DAY 8

THE MOST POWERFUL ANTI-CANCER FOODS

Three of the most powerful anti-cancer vegetables are garlic, leeks, and onions. Broccoli, Brussels sprouts, cauliflower, kale, red cabbage, curly cabbage, spinach, and beet root also have strong anti-cancer properties. Other noteworthy anti-cancer veggies include asparagus, green beans, radishes, and rutabaga.[2]

I concluded that the most efficient way to get the broadest array of anti-cancer nutrition into my body every day was to make Giant Salads and eat them for lunch and dinner. So that's what I did during the most intensive phase of my cancer-healing journey.

The Giant Salad is the simplest, most sustainable, most potent anti-cancer meal possible.

So what's the takeaway? Eat those vegetables! Throw them all in a bowl and make a Giant Salad. Add as many other veggies as you want. Add a little extra virgin olive oil and apple cider vinegar for dressing and enjoy.[3]

---

2 Yi-Fang Chu, Jie Sun, Xianzhong Wu, and Rui Hai Liu, "Antioxidant and Antiproliferative Activities of Common Vegetables," *Journal of Agriculture and Food Chemistry* 50, no. 23 (October 10, 2002): 6910–6916. https://doi.org/10.1021/jf020665f.
3 My entire anti-cancer dietary protocol is outlined in my book *Chris Beat Cancer: A Comprehensive Plan for Healing Naturally.*

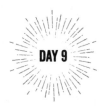

KEEP IT SIMPLE

Simple is sustainable. You must create a simple daily healing routine that you can stick with.

When I first adopted a raw food diet, I bought several recipe books with the fantasy of becoming a master of raw food. But I quickly figured out that menu planning, shopping for ingredients, and experimenting with new recipes every day would take a lot more time, energy, and effort than I had to spare. And many of these recipes wouldn't give me as much nutritional variety as a big bowl full of vegetables. That's as simple as it gets.

So I decided to eat Giant Salads for lunch and dinner every single day because I wanted to get as many anti-cancer vegetables into my body as possible at every meal.[4]

I knew I had to keep it simple or it wouldn't be sustainable.

You need as simple a strategy as possible.

Don't overcomplicate your routine. That just creates stress, which works against you. Gravitate toward simplicity in all things.

Today's Question: *How can I simplify?*

---

4 https://www.chrisbeatcancer.com/giantsalad

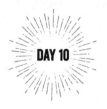

INTO THE CHRYSALIS

In order for a caterpillar to become a butterfly, it must withdraw from the world into a chrysalis (often called a cocoon, but a cocoon is for moths). Inside the chrysalis, the caterpillar's body breaks down into a liquid soup of imaginal cells, which rearrange themselves and solidify into a completely new body with different organs, long legs, antennae, and wings. Isn't that incredible?

Just like the caterpillar, you need to create the ideal conditions for your metamorphosis. You need to simplify your life as much as possible. You need peace and quiet. You need to insulate your mind and body from chaos, negativity, and stress. And you need plenty of time to rest, recover, and grow. You need *you time*. This is a season of seclusion, radical change, and lifelong transformation. Form a chrysalis around yourself during your healing season to nurture yourself and protect yourself as you transform so that you can one day emerge as a beautiful butterfly, spread your wings, and fly.

Today's Challenge: *What steps can you take to form a chrysalis around yourself?*

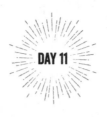

COMMIT YOUR WORKS TO THE LORD AND YOUR PLANS WILL BE ESTABLISHED.

—PROVERBS 16:3 (NASB)

COMMIT YOUR WAY TO THE LORD, TRUST ALSO IN HIM, AND HE WILL DO IT.

—PSALM 37:5 (NASB)

I commit my plans to you, Lord, and I trust that you will see them through and that you will make a way for me.

RELEARN EVERYTHING

Cancer means something went haywire. And many of the things you thought you knew about life and health may be wrong. Go ahead and assume everything you know is wrong. Of course, it isn't all wrong, but the only way to root out the wrongness is to reexamine it all.

This is a season of self-directed reeducation for you. Challenge all of your beliefs. Learn as much as possible.

Explore. Be curious. Consider every new idea and opinion, but don't be quick to jump to conclusions. Some ideas are powerfully seductive, shiny boxes with nothing inside.

Unpack them. Go deeper. Consider the sources. What are their motives? What are their incentives? Test what you are learning. Weigh the ideas against each other. Ruminate on them. Stew on them. Let them roll around in your head. Look for the common thread of truth that connects them together.

Always ask yourself, *Does this makes sense?* Listen to your instincts and intuition and to the Holy Spirit. Ask your Heavenly Father for wisdom and guidance. And don't forget to enjoy this season of learning and growth!

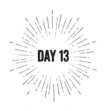

DAY 13

DOCUMENT YOUR JOURNEY

This may be the most challenging season of your life. You will be tested and stretched, refined, and pruned. It may be painful. But you will learn invaluable lessons that you can pass on to others. So get in the habit each day of writing things down. Don't trust your memory. Keep a notepad with you or make notes on your phone. Important things need to be recorded. Capture the details immediately and sort through them later.

Keep a journal. Write down your thoughts and fears and prayers. Write down what you do each day. Write down the memorable things people said to you and the things they did for you. Write down your answered prayers, the mini-miracles, the divine appointments, and the "coincidences." I'm telling you to do this because I wish I had done it more during the first two years of my cancer journey.

Record every conversation with your doctors and nurses on your phone. They will tell you important things you need to remember and may also say some surprising things you don't want to forget.

And make sure you ask the right questions. Use my free patient guide: *20 Questions for Your Oncologist*.

You can download it at www.chrisbeatcancer.com/20.

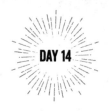

DAY 14

The 34th chapter of Psalms came alive to me after my cancer diagnosis. I hope these verses encourage you and ignite your faith as much as they did for me.

I sought the Lord, and he answered me;
*   he delivered me from all my fears.*

The eyes of the Lord are on the righteous,
*   and his ears are attentive to their cry;*

The righteous cry out, and the Lord hears them;
*   he delivers them from all their troubles.*

The righteous person may have many troubles,
*   but the Lord delivers him from them all.*

—Psalm 34:4,15,17,19 (NIV)

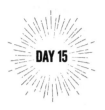

ALWAYS GET THREE BIDS

If you need to hire a contractor to work on your house, it's good practice to always get three bids. That way you can compare prices, professionalism, personalities, and check references in order to decide which contractor you want to work with.

If you pick the wrong person, they might do a sloppy job, take too long, leave the job unfinished, or run off with your money. Generally speaking, though, deciding who to hire to fix your house is a low-risk, low-stakes decision.

Deciding which doctor to hire to treat your cancer is a decision with the highest stakes possible, life or death. If they do a good job, you live. If they do a bad job, you die. You cannot afford to pick the wrong person.

So if you think it's wise to get three bids to paint your house, don't you think you should get at least three medical opinions on your cancer diagnosis and treatment options?

Don't let the first doctor you talk to rush you into treatment out of fear. You have time and you have more options than you realize. Get more advice and more opinions so you can make the best decision for you.

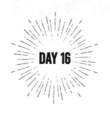

DAY 16

"FOR I WILL RESTORE YOU TO HEALTH, AND I WILL HEAL YOU OF YOUR WOUNDS," DECLARES THE LORD.

—JEREMIAH 30:17 (NASB)

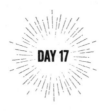

PHYSICAL THERAPY

You need 30 minutes of moderate to vigorous exercise a day, six days a week. Running, brisk walking, hiking, rebounding, cycling, cardio classes, weight training, Jazzercise, Zumba . . . any form of cardiovascular exercise is good for you.

Do not put exercise in the "whenever I get some free time" category. Daily exercise is mandatory physical therapy that turns off cancer-promoting genes and switches on anti-cancer genes in your body! Pick a time every day to exercise and block it off on your calendar. This is nonnegotiable.

If you have physical limitations, figure out what you *can* do and do it. If walking is all you can do, then walk for 20 to 30 minutes every day! No excuses.

Any kind of exercise that moves your body, increases your heart rate, and makes you break a sweat is wonderful. Just find something you enjoy and do it!

P.S. For some excuse-busting inspiration, google "Sean Stephenson Workout."

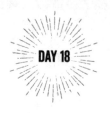

DAY 18

The Lord is my shepherd,
I shall not want.
He makes me lie down in green pastures;
He leads me beside quiet waters.
He restores my soul;
He guides me in the paths of righteousness
For His name's sake.
Even though I walk through the valley of the shadow of death,
I fear no evil, for You are with me;
Your rod and Your staff, they comfort me.
You prepare a table before me in the presence of my enemies;
You have anointed my head with oil;
My cup overflows.
Surely goodness and lovingkindness will follow me
all the days of my life,
And I will dwell in the house of the Lord forever.

—Psalm 23 (NASB)

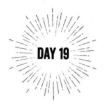

DAY 19

When Jesus came down from the mountain, large crowds followed Him. And a leper came to Him and bowed down before Him, and said, "Lord, if You are willing, You can make me clean." Jesus stretched out His hand and touched him, saying, "I am willing; be cleansed." And immediately his leprosy was cleansed.

—Matthew 8:1–3 (NASB)

Jesus Christ is the same yesterday, today, and forever (Hebrews 13:8). He is always willing to heal. The answer Jesus gave to the leper is the same one He gives to you.

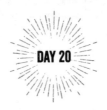

DAY 20

CANCER CHANGES EVERYTHING

I once heard a cancer patient say, "I'm not going to let cancer change me."

On the surface this may seem like an admirable pronouncement of strength and defiance toward the disease. But it is the wrong position to take.

Refusing to change is refusing to take responsibility for your situation. And that is a dangerous and powerless place to be.

Cancer will change you, like it or not.

So embrace it and let it change you for the better.

Let cancer be the wake-up call to change your whole life—to surrender and get right with God, to slow down, to simplify, to reorganize and reprioritize, to let go of things that don't serve you, to stop wasting precious time, to break your bad habits, to face down and conquer your fears, to take care of yourself like you never have before, to love and forgive the people who've hurt you, to be thankful for every day of life, and to become the best you you've ever been.

Today's Affirmation: *Cancer is changing me for the better.*

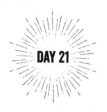

DAY 21

Specific instructions for those who need healing from the Apostle James in his letter to the church:

Is anyone among you suffering? Then he must pray.

Is anyone cheerful? He is to sing praises.

Is anyone among you sick? Then he must call for the elders of the church and they are to pray over him, anointing him with oil in the name of the Lord; and the prayer offered in faith will restore the one who is sick, and the Lord will raise him up, and if he has committed sins, they will be forgiven him.

Therefore, confess your sins to one another, and pray for one another so that you may be healed.

The effective prayer of a righteous man can accomplish much. Elijah was a man with a nature like ours, and he prayed earnestly that it would not rain, and it did not rain on the earth for three years and six months. Then he prayed again, and the sky poured rain and the earth produced its fruit.

—James 5:13–18 (NASB)

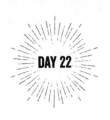

DAY 22

MASSIVE ACTION PRODUCES
MASSIVE RESULTS.

MINIMAL ACTION PRODUCES
MINIMAL RESULTS.

LET THE RESULTS YOU
WANT DETERMINE THE
KIND OF ACTION YOU TAKE.

I SUGGEST MASSIVE ACTION.

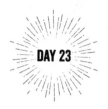

The purpose of a habit is to remove that action from self-negotiation. You no longer expend energy deciding whether to do it. You just do it. Good habits can range from telling the truth to flossing.

—Kevin Kelly

Here are some of the most important *Beat Cancer Daily* habits:

- Eating 10-plus servings of fruits and vegetables per day
- Juicing
- Exercising
- Spending time in the Bible
- Spending time in prayer and meditation
- Giving your fears and worries to God
- Practicing gratitude
- Choosing to think positively
- Forgiving everyone who has ever hurt you
- Forgiving new offenses quickly
- Getting eight or more hours of sleep each night

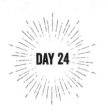

FORGIVENESS IS NOT A FEELING. IT'S A CHOICE.

If you're waiting until you "feel like it" to forgive someone, you may wait your entire lifetime!

In Luke 23:34 Jesus said, "Father, forgive them for they know not what they do." He said this while He was suffering immeasurable pain dying on a cross, innocent of any wrongdoing. Jesus was praying for His enemies from the most difficult circumstance imaginable, when He certainly didn't "feel like it."

Forgiveness is an act of love, and Jesus Christ showed us what love in action looks like by forgiving and praying for His enemies from the cross.

People have hurt you and they have hurt me. But those things pale in comparison to what was done to Jesus. If you're reading this, no one has crucified you. That's for sure!

If Jesus can forgive the people who nailed Him to a cross, then you and I have no excuse. We can and must forgive everyone who has ever hurt us.

Forgiveness is not a feeling. It's a choice. Your feelings will change after you make the decision to forgive.

Who do you need to forgive today?

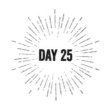

CAST YOUR CARES ON HIM

When my daughters were little, they loved to be helpful. One day while unloading groceries from the car, Mackenzie picked up a bag that was too heavy for her.

"Are you sure you've got it?" I said.

"Yep," she said confidently. But then after a few steps with it, she began to struggle and said, "Dad! I need help! It's too heavy!" And I quickly lifted the bag out of her arms.

Someone bigger than you, your Heavenly Father, wants to do that for you now.

God wants you to cast all of your cares onto Him (1 Peter 5:7). He wants you to give Him your heavy load: your worries, your fears, your problems. He wants to carry them for you because He loves you.

When you cast your cares onto God, you are letting go of them and saying, "I trust you."

One thing my daughter Mackenzie didn't do was ask me to give her back that heavy bag. Once I took it off her hands, she was done with it!

Cast your cares on Him. Trust your Heavenly Father with them. And don't pick them back up.

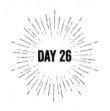

THE BATTLE

There is a battle involved in healing cancer, but it's not so much a battle in the body as it is a battle in the mind.

In order to heal your body, you must first win the battle in your mind. Changing your thoughts will change your life.

Fight fear and doubt with faith.

Believe you can get well.

Stop making excuses.

Take responsibility for your health.

Stop dwelling on the past.

Make plans for the future.

Forgive everyone, including yourself.

Choose positive thoughts.

Resist temptation.

Will yourself to action.

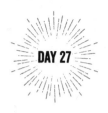

DAY 27

I WILL NOT DIE, BUT LIVE, AND DECLARE THE WORKS OF THE LORD.

—PSALM 118:17 (NKJV)

This is your motto now.

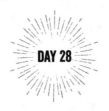

DON'T DEFER YOUR HOPE

Many of us use the word *hope* to express a wish or desire that something good will happen or that something bad won't happen. "I hope I get a promotion. . . . I hope I don't catch a cold. . . . I hope the dog doesn't pee in the house while I'm at work. . . . I hope this treatment cures me."

But the true expression of hope runs much deeper than wishful thinking. Hope is a desire coupled with a confident expectation that God is working even when we can't see it, because He loves us and is faithful.

Proverbs 13:12 says that hope deferred makes the heart grow sick. Notice it doesn't say "healing deferred" or "success deferred."

When we lose hope—the confidence that God is working everything out for our good—that's when discouragement, depression, despair, and hopelessness set in. That's when your heart becomes "sick." And a sick heart will produce a sick body. The antidote to this is to stop wishing and instead choose to believe that your Heavenly Father will supply all of your needs, and that He will heal you and deliver you from all of your fears.

False hope says, "I wish." True hope says, "I trust that God will."

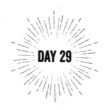

100 PERCENT IS EASY.
99 PERCENT IS HARD.

100 percent is not perfection.

100 percent is taking full responsibility for your life and health.

100 percent is total commitment.

100 percent is no excuses.

100 percent is being willing to change everything.

100 percent is taking Massive Action.

100 percent is letting go of the past.

100 percent is forgiving yourself.

100 percent is forgiving everyone else.

100 percent is believing you will succeed.

100 percent is refusing to doubt.

100 percent is trusting God with all of your heart.

100 percent is doing it when you don't feel like it.

100 percent is easy. 99 percent is hard.

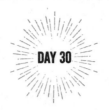

HEALING STRONG

"I am _____ ."

Years ago, when I was diagnosed with cancer, my answer was . . . *I am afraid. I am tired. I am sick. I am angry. I am a cancer patient.* . . .

Proverbs 18:21 says, "The tongue has the power of life and death, and those who love it will eat its fruit."

Your tongue has two functions: to feed your body and to feed your soul. What you put into your mouth can promote health and wellness, or it can promote disease and death. And what comes out of your mouth can do the same thing!

Your own words can build you up or tear you down. They can create an atmosphere of peace or one of disharmony. Your words can give hope or produce discouragement. They can be nourishing, life giving, and sweet or bitter, rotten, and poisonous.

Pay attention to the things you say to yourself and choose to speak words of life over your body and your situation.

My prayer for you today is that you will continually speak this over your life: I am healing strong!

—*Suzy Griswold, founder of HealingStrong*[5]

5   HealingStrong (healingstrong.org) is a nonprofit that helps to equip and empower cancer thrivers and others with life-giving connections and holistic education through local support groups.

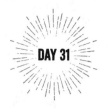

DAY 31

MAKE FEAR DISAPPEAR

You can run from your fears. You can avoid them. You can hide from them. You can pretend they don't exist. But the only way to get victory over your fears is to face them head-on. Lean into them. Advance against them. Beat them back. Crush them and conquer them.

Most fears are illusory, like a mirage in the desert. Move toward your fears and watch them disappear.

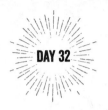

HEALING IS A MARATHON, NOT A SPRINT

In the modern world, where everything is at our fingertips, we have all developed a "quick fix" mentality. But chronic disease takes many years to develop.

There is no miracle cure or magic pill.

With the exception of miracles, you can't heal overnight.

Consistency is the key. Day by day, taking care of yourself, feeding your body food that promotes health, exercising, slowing down, removing harmful things . . .

All of this creates *healing momentum*.

Once you get the ball rolling, it's easier to keep it rolling.

That's why simplicity is important. Because simplicity is sustainable.

Pace yourself. And remember . . .

Slow and steady wins the race!

Healing is a marathon, not a sprint.

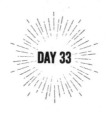

DAY 33

As [Jesus] was leaving Jericho with His disciples and a large crowd, a blind beggar named *Bartimaeus, the son of Timaeus, was sitting by the road.*

When he heard that it was Jesus the Nazarene, he began to cry out and say, "Jesus, Son of David, have mercy on me!"

Many were sternly telling him to be quiet, but he kept crying out all the more, "Son of David, have mercy on me!"

And Jesus stopped and said, "Call him here.*"*

So they called the blind man, saying to him, "Take courage, stand up! He is calling for you." Throwing aside his cloak, he jumped up and came to Jesus.

And answering him, Jesus said, "What do you want Me to do for you?"

And the blind man said to Him, "Rabboni (my Master), I want *to regain my sight!"*

And Jesus said to him, "Receive your sight; your faith has made you well." Immediately he regained his sight and began *following Him, glorifying God; and when all the people saw it, they gave praise to God.*

—MARK 10:46–51, LUKE 18:42–43 (NASB)

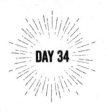

TIME TO SAY NO

Saying yes is exciting. It makes you feel good. It also means you don't have to disappoint anyone, which is often why we do it, because saying no can be awkward and uncomfortable.

I love saying yes to new things and new experiences. But saying yes has a downside. It distracts you from your focus. Always saying yes creates too much work, too many obligations, too many commitments, and too many responsibilities.

When I said yes to writing two more books for my publisher (you're reading one of them now), it required a huge commitment of time, energy, and effort. In order to accomplish this, I had to say no to a lot of other things that I also wanted to do.

Say yes to things that support your goals, further your mission, and serve your purpose. Say yes to the things that are most important right now. And say no to everything else.

If you have cancer, healing should be a top priority. And in order to devote the time and effort necessary to heal, you need to create more space in your life and reduce your stress by saying no to many of the things you used to say yes to. It's time to say no.

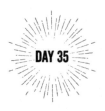

DAY 35

Healing is a creative act calling for all the hard work and dedication needed for other forms of creativity.

—BERNIE SIEGEL, M.D., FROM *LOVE, MEDICINE AND MIRACLES*

Creation requires action. Action means there is work involved.

Artists work to create art. They paint. They play guitar. They write. They design. They build. . . .

The work produces a result.

People become artists because they enjoy creating. They enjoy the work—the creative process—not just the reward that the finished product provides.

You are creating health each day with your choices and your actions.

You are building a new body. There is work involved. But it's worth it. Choose to enjoy the creative healing work you are doing today.

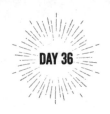

DAY 36

FORGIVENESS IS NOT AN EMOTION. . . . FORGIVENESS IS AN ACT OF THE WILL, AND THE WILL CAN FUNCTION REGARDLESS OF THE TEMPERATURE OF THE HEART.

—CORRIE TEN BOOM

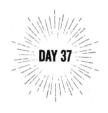

DON'T FEAR THE FUTURE

The fear of what could be is almost always worse than the reality of what is.

Anxiety, worry, fear for the future, and fear of the unknown are our biggest sources of stress.

Step 1: Decide not to worry about the future and give your fears and worries to God today and every day. Trust Him with your life and your future. There's a promise in Jeremiah 29:11 for you:

> *"For I know the plans I have for you," declares the*
> *Lord, "plans to prosper you and not to harm you. Plans*
> *to give you hope and a future."*

Step 2: When you catch yourself worrying about the future, repeat Step 1!

Practically speaking, you're better off knowing what you're dealing with than not knowing. Deliberately not knowing often produces excessive and unnecessary fear and anxiety.

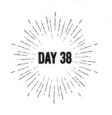

DAY 38

EVERYTHING IN LIFE HAPPENS FOR A REASON . . . AND MOST OF THE TIME THE REASON IS YOU.

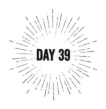

DON'T LET LITTLE THINGS GET IN THE WAY OF BIG THINGS

Sometimes it's easy to be distracted by little details that seem important in the moment but, in the grand scheme of things, are not important at all.

Uncertainty and unanswered questions about little things can lead to "analysis paralysis" and become excuses that prevent you from taking action. And when no action is taken, nothing happens, and nothing changes.

There are unknowns on every journey. There's no way to be completely prepared. You will learn and grow and figure things out as you go. Things will get easier and you will get better at it. If you find yourself feeling tripped up over something, ask yourself: *Is this a little thing or a big thing?*

Don't let little things get in the way of big things.

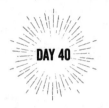

MAKE YOUR BED

If you want to change the world, start off by making your bed.

*If you make your bed every morning, you will
have accomplished the first task of the day.*

*It will give you a small sense of pride, and it will encourage
you to do another task and another and another.*

*And by the end of the day, that one task completed
will have turned into many tasks completed.*

*Making your bed will also reinforce the
fact that the little things in life matter.*

*If you can't do the little things right, you'll
never be able to do the big things right.*

*And if by chance you have a miserable day, you will come
home to a bed that is made—that you made—and a made
bed gives you encouragement that tomorrow will be better.*

—ADMIRAL WILLIAM H. MCRAVEN[6]

6   Admiral William H. McRaven, commencement address to the graduates of the University of Texas at Austin on May 17, 2014. https://jamesclear.com/great-speeches/make-your-bed-by-admiral-william-h-mcraven.

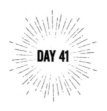

DAY 41

Choose not to be harmed—and you won't feel harmed.
Don't feel harmed—and you haven't been.

—MARCUS AURELIUS

We often forget, or perhaps many of us were never taught, that being offended is a choice. And that you can actually choose not to be harmed by the words and actions of others. It's simply a matter of not letting your emotions rule you. The world is full of bickering, fighting, rudeness, offensiveness, and outrage. Don't take anything personally, including personal attacks. Don't respond and don't jump into the mud pit. Choose not to be harmed and fly above it.

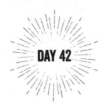

DON'T WORRY ABOUT TOMORROW

Jesus Christ gives good advice. In Matthew 6:34 (NIV) He says, "Do not worry about tomorrow, for tomorrow will worry about itself. Each day has enough trouble of its own." Jesus said, "Don't worry about tomorrow." So, don't worry about tomorrow! You can only handle one moment at a time, and one day at a time. Just focus on right now, on today's tasks, today's challenges, and today's to-do list.

You can and should make plans for tomorrow, and for the future. But you should not let all the "what-ifs" and the infinite number of calamities that you can imagine create fear, worry, and anxiety in your mind and in your heart.

Worry is a bad habit. And you can break it! When fear starts to creep in, you can either let your mind and emotions run wild, or you can choose to give your fear to God and not worry. Don't worry about tomorrow.

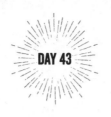

DAY 43

NO ONE WILL TAKE BETTER CARE OF YOU THAN YOU, IF YOU CHOOSE TO.

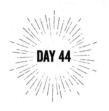

DAY 44

You are what you eat, drink, breathe, think, say and do.

—Patricia Bragg

You are what you eat. The nutrients from whole unprocessed food nourish your body, feed your cells, and become a part of you, changing your body for the better. But that's only half the equation.

Cancer gives you the opportunity to change not just what you eat, but who you are—the person you are inside your body.

Changing the way you think, speak, and act changes who you are. So what kind of person are you? Are you negative, critical, judgmental, impatient, selfish, resentful, or worrisome? If you have any of these tendencies, I have good news! You can become more patient, kind, and loving, more like Jesus.

This is a season of self-improvement. Step by step, day by day, you will improve your diet, improve your environment, improve your thoughts, improve your words, and improve your actions.

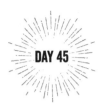

HOW MANY TIMES SHOULD YOU FORGIVE?

Then Peter came and said to him, "Lord, how often shall my brother sin against me and I forgive him? Up to seven times?" Jesus said to him, "I do not say to you, up to seven times, but up to seventy times seven."

—MATTHEW 18:21–22 (NIV)

Seventy times seven is 490 times. Did Jesus mean that 490 times is the absolute limit, and that you should keep a running tally of offenses for each person in your life, and when they hit number 491, you officially have permission to not forgive them? Of course not. Our Heavenly Father continues to forgive us, so we should continue to forgive others.

The Lord is slow to anger, abounding in love and forgiving every kind of sin and rebellion.

—Numbers 14:18 (NIV)

Jesus's point was to keep forgiving. Forgiveness is a mental, emotional, and spiritual action that protects your heart, soul, and body from being poisoned by bitterness.

Forgiveness does not make the offense okay, and it does not mean you must continue to endure abuse from someone. If there are people in your life who continue to hurt you, you need to get away from them. And you also need to forgive them.

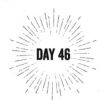

CHEW ON THIS

Today I have some practical advice on how to extract the most nutrition from your food.

Chew it better.

Many of us assume that digestion happens in the stomach, but the digestive process actually starts in your mouth. The grinding action of your teeth and the enzymes in your saliva work together to break down each bite and extract the vital nutrients from it. The better you chew your food, the more nutrition you absorb after you swallow.

Most of us eat mindlessly.

Today I want you to practice "conscious mindful eating" and chew each bite thoroughly. Crush it, pulverize it, and completely liquify it before you swallow. Some hardcore health advocates recommend 100 chews per mouthful. Now, that is a lot! I suggest at least 30 chews per bite. Yes, it takes longer to eat. But it's worth it.

It takes about 20 minutes for your stomach to tell your brain that you are full. If you are trying to lose weight, thoroughly chewing each bite will prevent you from overeating and will naturally reduce your calorie consumption at each meal.

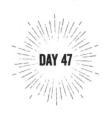

DAY 47

GOD IS OUR REFUGE AND STRENGTH, ALWAYS READY TO HELP IN TIMES OF TROUBLE.

—PSALM 46:1 (NLT)

Father, thank you that you are my refuge and strength. Thank you that you are always ready to help me whenever I am in trouble!

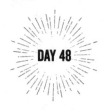

JUST CHUG IT

Vegetables and I are not the best of friends. I have taste and texture issues. But after a diagnosis of Hodgkin's lymphoma at 26, I made the choice to heal my body with nutrition and nontoxic therapies rather than undergo chemotherapy. And to my dismay, I learned that the most potent anti-cancer foods are vegetables!

If there was a way to get broccoli, Brussels sprouts, cauliflower, and cabbage into my body with a feeding tube, I would have done it. But that wasn't an option. So I made a giant veggie smoothie, thinking that would be easier.

The first sip made me gag. So did the second sip. And the third. The only way I could get it down was to hold my nose. I told myself, *Just chug it!* And I did chug it, like my life depended on it. Every single day for seven years, I held my nose and chugged a 64-ounce veggie smoothie. And along the way, my body healed itself! Even today, 12 years later, I still drink this smoothie at least four times a week!

I want to encourage you with all of my heart and cheerleading skills to *do hard things!* You are worth it! Food is medicine. Even if you have to pinch your nose, do whatever it takes to get nutritious life-saving food into your body every day. Just chug it!

—*Cortney Campbell*[7]

7   Cortney Campbell is a holistic Hodgkin's lymphoma survivor. Connect with her at www.anticancermom.com.

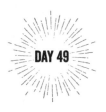

REMOVE FRICTION

We all need a little friction in life to smooth our rough edges and to sharpen us. But too much friction can slow you down, wear you down, and even grind you to a halt.

Friction makes things difficult when they don't need to be.

In practical terms, friction is the unnecessary steps, extra time, and mental or physical energy you have to expend every time you want to do something. Friction makes it a drag.

In January 2003 I decided to start drinking 64 ounces of vegetable juice every day. I could either run the juicer six to eight times per day and drink the freshest juice possible or I could make the entire batch in the morning and drink it throughout the day. I chose the latter because it was sustainable, with the least amount of friction. Later I learned that the nutritional difference was negligible.

Now is the time to simplify your life and remove the things (or people) that are causing unnecessary friction.

Today's Challenge: *Think about the areas where you are feeling friction and ask yourself:* What is making this feel hard? What could I change or remove to make this easier?

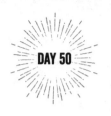

DAY 50

TO BE CONSCIOUS THAT YOU ARE IGNORANT IS A GREAT STEP TO KNOWLEDGE.

—BENJAMIN DISRAELI

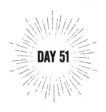

BODY BUILDING

Your body is made up of trillions of cells, and most of your soft tissue and organs are replaced and rebuilt every three months. Your body is made of the food you eat, the water you drink, and the air you breathe. That's it.

You built your body.

You are what you ate.

Your body is a perpetual construction site. Exercise sends survival signals to your body to rebuild itself stronger and more fit. And the food you eat supplies the raw materials that your body needs to repair, regenerate, and detoxify.

You have the power every day to build yourself a better body with exercise and nutrient-rich food from the earth.

Every time you sit down to eat, think to yourself, *I am building a new body.*

And if you are tempted to eat something you know you shouldn't, an easy way to overcome the temptation is to ask yourself this simple question: *Is this food promoting health or disease in my body?*

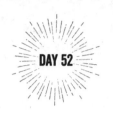

DAY 52

FORGIVENESS IS LIKE A HEALTHY DIET. IT ONLY WORKS IF YOU STICK WITH IT.

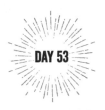

DAY 53

WHEN TO EAT, WHEN NOT TO EAT . . .

Today I want to encourage you to eat all of your meals in an 11-hour window. This gives you 13 hours of nightly fasting. Late-night eating is a really bad habit that interferes with the incredible restorative benefits of sleep and eventually wrecks your health. That's why it's best to go to bed on an empty stomach.

If you start eating breakfast at 8 A.M., finish dinner by 7 P.M. or earlier. If you eat breakfast earlier than 8 A.M., you should eat dinner earlier. Or you could eat two meals: a late breakfast, a late lunch, and no dinner.

Do not skip breakfast and only eat lunch and dinner.

Your body processes food most efficiently early in the day. Breakfast and lunch should be your largest meals.

This simple practice of "time-restricted feeding" has been found to increase weight loss and reduce blood pressure, inflammation, insulin resistance, blood sugar, and oxidative stress. You may also find that you have more energy during the day and sleep better at night.

One study found that breast cancer patients who fasted for less than 13 hours per night had a 36 percent higher risk of recurrence than those who fasted for 13 hours or more.[8] Eating in an 8-hour window with up to 16 hours of nightly fasting could be even more beneficial, especially if you have weight you want to lose.

---

8   Marinac et al., "Prolonged Nightly Fasting and Breast Cancer Prognosis," *JAMA Oncology* 2, no. 8 (August 1, 2016): 1049–1055.

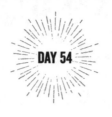

DAY 54

IN ALL THINGS WE SHOULD TRY TO MAKE OURSELVES BE AS GRATEFUL AS POSSIBLE.

—SENECA

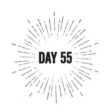

A PRAYER OF THANKSGIVING AND GRATITUDE FOR YOUR BODY

I will give thanks to You, for I am fearfully and
wonderfully made; Wonderful are Your works,
And my soul knows it very well.

—Psalm 139:14 (NASB)

Thank you, God, for my body.

Thank you for my eyes and my ears. Thank you for my nose, my mouth, my teeth, and my tongue.

Thank you for my arms and my legs, my hands and my feet, my fingers and my toes.

Thank you for my brain, my heart, my liver, and my lungs. Thank you for my pancreas, my spleen, my gallbladder, and my digestive tract. Thank you for my muscles and my bones. Thank you for my immune system. My cardiovascular system. My nervous system. Thank you for my blood.

Thank you for my skin. Thank you for my hair. Thank you for every cell in my body. Thank you that I am fearfully and wonderfully made!

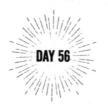

DAY 56

Be still, and know that I am God.
—Psalm 46:10 (NIV)

This verse comes with an assignment. Block off at least five minutes on your calendar every day and make time to be still.

Find a quiet, comfortable place to sit. Set a five-minute timer on your phone. Close your eyes. Relax your body. Focus on your breath. Breath is life. Living things breathe.

Breathe in and out through your nose. Inhale deeply and exhale slowly in a controlled manner, like slowly letting air out of a balloon. Your inhale and your exhale should take the same amount of time, but your exhale may be longer.

As you inhale, pay attention to your breath and your body. Feel the life-giving air flowing into your nose and filling up your lungs. As you exhale, listen to the sound your breath makes as you release it from your body. Feel your lungs deflate and relax. Feel your heart beat between breaths. Take at least 10 deep breaths this way.

During these few minutes of stillness, just be with your Creator, your Heavenly Father. You can pray and talk to Him or meditate on Scripture or just be still and enjoy God's goodness, His peace that surpasses all understanding, and His presence in your life. Know that He is in control. That He cares about you and will supply all of your needs.

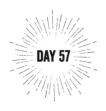

A PEACEFUL, QUIET LIFE

This is the goal. To live a peaceful, quiet life that is conducive to health and healing. Now, your life may not always be quiet, especially if you have young children or a dog like mine that barks at everything that moves. But you can still have peace.

Is there too much noise in your life? By noise I mean anything that causes chaos, confusion, disharmony, anxiety, and stress. Are there noisy things in your life causing you stress that you can remove?

Some examples of stress-producing noise are the news and social media, negative people, and an overwhelming number of commitments and responsibilities.

Removing the noise from your life leaves space for a more peaceful, quiet life.

You have the permission, freedom, and power to remove stressful things from your life.

Don't put this off. Have some conversations, make some calls, send some emails, delete some apps, unplug from as much stress-producing noise as fast as you can, and create for yourself a more peaceful, quiet life.

YOU HAVE

Cancer taught me—and I hope it's teaching you—what was really important in life. Before cancer, I was chasing happiness and I took much of my life for granted. Then cancer gave me a hard reset. And during my healing season, I found so much joy in the things I had never fully appreciated—fruits and vegetables, nature, fresh air, sunshine, mobility, freedom, family, and a relationship with my Heavenly Father. Choose to be happy, give thanks, celebrate, and enjoy what you have right now. You have everything you need for life and godliness (2 Peter 1:3). You have more than enough.

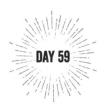

ASSUME THE POWER POSITION

One of the most powerful things you can say is . . .

"This is my fault."

Humans don't like to be at fault. Because fault and mistakes imply inferiority, weakness, and stupidity. This is why we like to blame others.

But when we blame our problems on others or on bad luck, we become a victim.

As I say often, *"Everything in life happens for a reason . . . and most of the time, the reason is you."*

Is every problem in your life 100 percent your fault? Of course not.

But believing that *nothing* is ever your fault puts you in a position of denial, weakness, and victimhood.

Taking personal responsibility, without beating yourself up for your mistakes, is taking a position of strength and power over your problems. When you do this, you also activate the creative problem-solving part of your brain to help you find a solution to your problems.

The victim says, "I can't."

The problem solver asks, "How can I?"

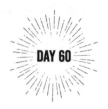

HOW TO FORGIVE YOURSELF

I've often heard people say, "The hardest person to forgive is yourself." It is hard, and if you are struggling with forgiving yourself, hopefully these thoughts will make it easier. Guilt and shame from your past are powerfully destructive emotions. They are just as toxic as bitterness and resentment toward others. Forgiveness frees you from guilt and shame. But you may not feel worthy of forgiveness.

If you've ever been hired or promoted, you may remember feeling unworthy of your new title. But you had to accept your new identity, embrace your new reality, and start acting like a manager, a director, a boss, whatever . . . or else you wouldn't last long in that position.

John 1:9 (NASB) says, "If we confess our sins, He is faithful and just to forgive us our sins and to cleanse us from all unrighteousness."

Your Heavenly Father loves you, sees you as worthy, and is willing to forgive you as soon as you ask. So ask for forgiveness, accept it knowing that it's done, and embrace your new reality: forgiven with a clean slate.

Once you know your Heavenly Father has forgiven you, there's no reason you can't forgive yourself.

Father, thank you for forgiving me and cleansing me from all unrighteousness. Thank you for your unfailing love. Because you have forgiven me, I forgive myself.

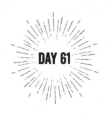

DAY 61

ONLY ONE WHO ATTEMPTS THE ABSURD IS CAPABLE OF ACHIEVING THE IMPOSSIBLE.

—MIGUEL DE UNAMUNO

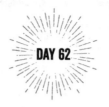

DAY 62

BE BOLD

Have confidence in yourself. Do not be afraid. Fear does not stop death; it steals life and prevents peace. No amount of worry has ever cured any disease.

Cancer first comes as an oppressor, but if you let it, cancer will become your teacher. The lessons it brings are beautiful and wondrous gifts. Indescribable. Unexpected. And perfect.

Take this as an opportunity to reset, recalibrate, and redefine what living really is. Look forward to your life after cancer. What gifts will you pass on to others? How will you inspire them? Be ready to tell your story. It has the power to change another person's life.

Now ask yourself, *How can I live my life differently? Where have I been small? Where have I been absent? How can I take better care of myself? Do I want to survive or thrive?*

Choose to be a thriver. Let go of what was and embrace what will be. Let your suffering turn into something beautiful for yourself and for others.

This is your moment to *heal*. You are worthy and you are worth fighting for!

—Kim Hanson, breast cancer survivor[9]

9 Connect with Kim and Theo Hanson at www.thevidacenter.com.

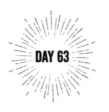

DO THE CAN-DOS

Don't get discouraged by what you can't do. Focus on what you *can do, and do those things.*

Do the can-dos now. And chip away at the can't-dos along the way.

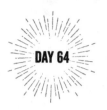

DAY 64

THE ULTIMATE MULTITASKING EXERCISE ROUTINE

Here's how to supercharge the benefits of your exercise routine:

- Exercise outside, exposing as much of your body to the sun as possible to increase your vitamin D levels and improve your immune function.

- Listen to healing Scriptures or healing-frequency music, or sing along to worship music while you exercise.

- Take at least 10 deep breaths of fresh air before, during, and after you exercise to increase oxygen in your body.

- Exercise vigorously enough to get sweaty, which increases detoxification.

- Spend a few minutes in prayer, meditation, and affirmations when you finish exercising to calm your nervous system and reduce stress.

- All this can be done in as little as 30 minutes. I suggest 20 to 30 minutes of exercise and then 10 to 20 minutes of cool-down with prayer, meditation, and affirmations.

- Think about what other health-promoting activities you can combine.

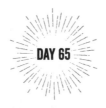

ENCOURAGEMENT FROM PSALM 91

Whoever dwells in the shelter of the Most High will rest in the shadow of the Almighty. I will say of the Lord, "He is my refuge and my fortress, my God, in whom I trust."

Surely He will save you from the fowler's snare and from the deadly pestilence. He will cover you with his feathers, and under his wings you will find refuge; his faithfulness will be your shield and rampart. . . .

If you say, "The Lord is my refuge," and you make the Most High your dwelling, no harm will overtake you, no disaster will come near your tent. For he will command his angels concerning you to guard you in all your ways; they will lift you up in their hands, so that you will not strike your foot against a stone.

"Because he loves me," says the Lord, "I will rescue him; I will protect him, for he acknowledges My name. He will call on me, and I will answer him; I will be with him in trouble, I will deliver him and honor him. With long life I will satisfy him and show him My salvation."

—Psalm 91:1–4,9–12,14–16 (NIV)

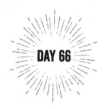

YOU DON'T HAVE TO BE WHO YOU WERE

"I am who I am." No, you are who you choose to be.

Time and circumstances change people, sometimes for the worse. And if somewhere along the way you became someone you don't like or other people don't like, that's okay. Because you're not an old dog. You can learn some new tricks. You can change!

Every day is an opportunity to choose to be the person you want to be, the person God created you to be, the person you were destined to be . . . the best you possible. The greatest you in the history of you!

You can't fix a problem doing the same things that caused it.

If the person you used to be got you into the mess that you're in, then it's time to give yourself a reboot. Delete some bad programs and install a new operating system.

Challenges in life are often the catalyst for change. They force us to rise up and be more than we thought we could be.

You can be more loving, more generous, more kind, more patient, more disciplined, more organized, more responsible, more thoughtful. . . . You don't have to be who you were.

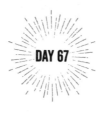

DAY 67

The fear of the Lord is the beginning of wisdom, and the knowledge of the Holy One is understanding. For by me your days will be multiplied, and years of life will be added to you.

—Proverbs 9:10–11 (NASB)

There are two kinds of fear: the good kind and the bad kind.

The fear of the Lord isn't the stress-producing kind of fear, like the fear of cancer or the fear of a villain or a monster in a scary movie. It's actually a healthy, positive kind of fear.

Fear the Lord in the same way you would fear a king who is also your father.

Fearing the Lord is maintaining an attitude of love and reverence for your Heavenly Father, with submission to Him as the Creator and King of the Universe and righteous judge of all things.

The fear of displeasing Him, being out of favor with Him, being separated from Him, and the eternal consequences of living a life of rebellion against Him compels us to surrender, trust, and obey. And fearing the Lord has benefits! His promise of wisdom, protection, healing, blessings, and extra years of life!

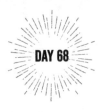

REDUCE YOUR TOXIC LOAD

Your body is always detoxifying whenever you sweat, pee, poop, and exhale.

Your body is able to detoxify much faster when you stop polluting it with alcohol, tobacco, and drugs; artificial additives, preservatives, flavors, colors, sweeteners, and trans fats in processed food; pesticides, fungicides, and herbicides sprayed on conventionally grown produce; and saturated fat, heme iron, antibiotics, viruses, parasites, and pathogens found in animal-based food.

Here are the biggest levers to dramatically reduce your toxic load:

- Stop using tobacco and alcohol.
- Get off pharmaceuticals as much as possible with your doctor's help.
- Switch to a plant-based diet (as organic as possible).
- Filter your water to remove chlorine, fluoride, and other contaminants.
- Replace your body-care products with organic or nontoxic brands.
- Replace your home-cleaning products with organic or nontoxic brands.

Note: Produce with thin skin is more apt to absorb pesticides than produce with thicker skin. If you eat the skin, buy organic. If you don't eat the skin, conventional may be okay.

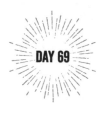

COME TO ME, ALL WHO ARE
WEARY AND HEAVY-LADEN,
AND I WILL GIVE YOU REST. TAKE MY
YOKE UPON YOU AND LEARN FROM
ME, FOR I AM GENTLE AND HUMBLE IN
HEART, AND YOU WILL FIND REST FOR
YOUR SOULS. FOR MY YOKE IS EASY
AND MY BURDEN IS LIGHT.

—JESUS
—MATTHEW 11:28–30 (NASB)

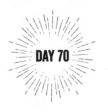

A THOUSAND THINGS

My daughters live in a bubble. All their needs are met. They have nothing to complain about, but of course they still do (they are children, after all). One day, my daughter Mackenzie was sitting next to me at the kitchen counter pouting about something that didn't go her way, something so utterly insignificant that I can't remember what it was.

I have an extremely low tolerance for complaining from my kids, and in a moment of frustration I blurted out something that was accidentally profound. I turned to her and sternly said, "You have a thousand things to be happy about. Pick one."

She got quiet. I could see her mind working. And almost instantly, her attitude changed. And I thought to myself, *Wow. That was pretty good!*

Nearly every day, things come our way that try to steal our happiness and distract us from the countless blessings we have. I had a lot to be unhappy about in 2004. My wife and I were in a tiny house, struggling financially, and I had cancer.

But that's when I learned that gratitude is the secret to happiness. In any difficult circumstance, it just takes a moment to count your blessings and thank God for them. This will reset your perspective and stir up thankfulness and joy in your heart.

No matter what life throws at you, remember: You have a thousand things to be happy about. Pick one.

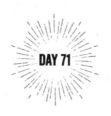

DAY 71

IF YOU ARE HAVING A HARD TIME FORGIVING YOURSELF AND YOU FEEL LIKE YOU DESERVE TO BE PUNISHED, COULD WE CALL IT TIME SERVED?

—BROOKE GOLDNER, M.D.

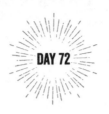

DAY 72

Critical, cynical, negative people notice every flaw and every problem in every situation. That used to be me. But cancer taught me that in any situation I could look for the positive, the bright side, the silver lining.

Many blessings come disguised as problems. When things don't go your way—when plans go haywire and you're feeling frustrated, disappointed, discouraged, and depressed—take a moment to step back and consider, *Maybe good will come from this. Maybe this is a blessing in disguise.*

You don't have to pretend a bad thing is good. But instead, put your mind to work and imagine the good things that could come out of the bad situation. That will reframe the present and shift your perspective toward the future.

Here's how I exercise my faith in response to problems and "bad things."

First, I remind myself of Romans 8:28 (NIV), which says that "God works all things for the good of those who love Him, who have been called according to his purpose."

Second, I respond with a simple prayer of faith: *Father, thank you that you will work this for my good because I love you, and I know I am called according to your purpose.*

Third, I vocalize my faith. When discussing my problem, I say something like, "You know what? This situation stinks. I don't like it. But I know that God is going to work this out for my good. Something good will come from this."

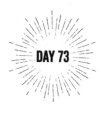

A merry heart does good, like medicine,
But a broken spirit dries the bones.

—PROVERBS 17:22 (NKJV)

A merry heart is a joyful, cheerful, happy heart. So you need to make it a point to laugh every single day.

Turn off the news, reality shows, dramas, and conflict, and focus on the things that bring laughter and joy into your life.

Quit being so serious. Let loose. Goof around. Make jokes. Retell funny stories. Be a kid again. Be silly! Be ridiculous!

Spend time with people who bring you joy, and make an effort to make the people around you smile and laugh.

Attend laughter therapy classes, read humorous books, watch sitcoms or stand-up comedy, or do all of the above to give yourself a dose of immune-boosting laughter medicine every single day.

A merry heart will do you good, like medicine!

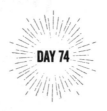

NEVER GIVE UP

God is faithful, who will not allow you to be tempted beyond what you are able, but with the temptation will also provide the way of escape.

—1 Corinthians 10:13 (NASB)

At age 45, I heard the dreaded words: *"It's cancer."* I was given three to six months to live unless I had more surgery, aggressive chemo, and radiation. But I took the time I needed to learn *why* I got cancer, and what cancer is. I met with doctors, talked with cancer patients, and tirelessly researched conventional and alternative cancer treatments.

I discovered God-given ways to treat my entire person—body, soul, and spirit. Techniques that attack the root causes of disease, not just the symptoms. Was I tempted to give up? Sure. Did I second-guess my choices? Of course. Did I get worse before I got better? Yes. But I never gave up. Ultimately, with hard work and consistent effort, my immune system completely eliminated the cancer naturally—without chemotherapy, radiation, or additional surgery. God led me to a Scripture at the beginning of my journey that gave me strength to keep learning and fighting, and to never give up.

Overcome the temptation to quit. If you've been knocked down, get back up. Don't stop fighting until you win.

—*Paula Black, author of* Life, Cancer and God[10]

---

10 Watch my interview Paula Black at http://www.chrisbeatcancer.com/paulablack.

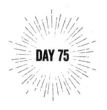

DAY 75

Be anxious for nothing, but in everything by prayer and supplication with thanksgiving, let your requests be made known to God. And the peace of God, which surpasses all comprehension, will guard your hearts and your minds in Christ Jesus.

—PHILIPPIANS 4:6–7 (NASB)

Don't worry about anything. Instead, pray.

Consciously give all of your worries and fears to God, thanking Him for all the good things in your life and trusting Him to supply all of your needs.

When you do this, He will give you peace in your heart and in your mind and a sense of calm in the middle of whatever storm surrounds you.

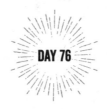

THE #1 ANTI-CANCER VITAMIN

In 2016 a landmark study found that women over 55 with blood concentrations of vitamin D_3 higher than 40 ng/ml had a 67 percent lower risk of cancer than women with levels lower than 20 ng/ml. The researchers concluded that optimal levels for cancer prevention are between 40 and 60 ng/ml, and that most cancers occur in people with vitamin D blood levels between 10 and 40 ng/ml.[11]

The best source of vitamin D_3 is sunshine. Ten to twenty minutes of sun on your skin per day, without sunscreen, is recommended. But the amount of D_3 you can get from the sun varies on the basis of your age, your BMI, your skin tone, your location, the season, the weather, and genetic factors.

Supplementing with 1,000 to 10,000 IU of D_3 per day is the easiest solution. I take more in the winter than in the summer.

Today's Action Step: *Have your D_3 levels checked by your doctor or at a walk-in blood lab and supplement accordingly.*

Note: Magnesium increases D_3 absorption and D_3 increases calcium absorption. Vitamin K_2 helps your body use calcium appropriately. It may be helpful to supplement magnesium and K_2, along with D_3.[12]

---

11 McDonnell et al., "Serum 25-Hydroxyvitamin D Concentrations ≥40 ng/ml Are Associated with >65% Lower Cancer Risk: Pooled Analysis of Randomized Trial and Prospective Cohort Study," *PLOS One* 11, no. 4 (April 6, 2016): e0152441. https://journals.plos.org/plosone/article?id=10.1371/journal.pone.0152441
12 Read this blog post for more information: https://www.chrisbeatcancer.com/vitamin-d-the-1-anti-cancer-vitamin/.

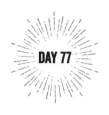

DAY 77

A GOOD LAUGH
AND A LONG SLEEP
ARE THE BEST CURES IN
THE DOCTOR'S BOOK.

—IRISH PROVERB

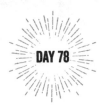

THE STORY OF ASA, KING OF JUDAH

In the thirty-ninth year of his reign, Asa was afflicted with a disease in his feet. Though his disease was severe, even in his illness he did not seek help from the Lord but only from the physicians. Then in the forty-first year of his reign Asa died and rested with his ancestors.

—2 Chronicles 16:12–13 (NIV)

Asa was a king who honored God during his reign, and as a result, the nation of Judah was blessed with peace and prosperity. But later in life, Asa developed a foot disease, and he didn't seek the Lord. He took his problem to physicians who couldn't help him, and he ended up dying from it.

Take your problems to God first. Put your faith, hope, and trust in Him above everything else. Doctors, treatments, nutrition, and exercise all have their place. But make sure you are seeking the help and direction of your Heavenly Father. He will direct your steps and lead you in the path of healing![13]

---

13 The story of King Asa can be found in 2 Chronicles 14–16.

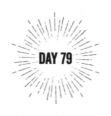

DAY 79

IF YOU HAVE A SICK HEART, YOU'RE GOING TO HAVE A SICK BODY.

FORGIVENESS HEALS YOUR HEART.

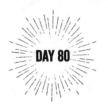

LIVE FOR TOMORROW

I eat healthy today because I want to be healthy tomorrow.

I exercise today because I want to be fitter and stronger tomorrow.

I organize today because I want to be organized tomorrow.

I save and invest money today because I want to be wealthier tomorrow.

I give generously today because I want to receive generously tomorrow.

I am loving and kind today because I want to enjoy love and kindness tomorrow.

I show mercy today because I want to be shown mercy tomorrow.

I forgive today because I want to be forgiven tomorrow.

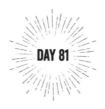

In Mark 9, a man brings his son, who is possessed by an evil spirit, to Jesus:

> *When the spirit saw Jesus, it immediately threw the boy into a convulsion. He fell to the ground and rolled around, foaming at the mouth. Jesus asked the boy's father, "How long has he been like this?"*
>
> *"From childhood," he answered. "It has often thrown him into fire or water to kill him. But if you can do anything, take pity on us and help us."*
>
> *"If you can?" said Jesus. "Everything is possible for one who believes."*
>
> *Immediately the boy's father exclaimed, "I do believe; help me overcome my unbelief!"*
>
> *When Jesus saw that a crowd was running to the scene, He rebuked the impure spirit. "You deaf and mute spirit," he said, "I command you, come out of him and never enter him again." The spirit shrieked, convulsed him violently and came out. The boy looked so much like a corpse that many said, "He's dead." But Jesus took him by the hand and lifted him to his feet, and he stood up.*
>
> —Mark 9:20–27 (NIV)

If you are struggling with faith and doubt, ask God to help you overcome your unbelief. He will!

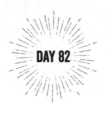
DAY 82

EVERY DAY MAY NOT BE GOOD, BUT THERE'S SOMETHING GOOD IN EVERY DAY.

—ALICE MORSE EARLE

Look for the good in today.

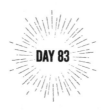

THE SECRET TO HAPPINESS

When I was diagnosed with cancer, I had a lot of things to be unhappy about. But I realized I could either focus on the bad things in my life or I could focus on the good things.

If you focus on the negative, it makes you miserable. But when you focus on the good things in your life, it brings you joy and gratitude. In my most difficult season of life, I learned to shift my focus from the things I wasn't happy about—the things that were frustrating me, scaring me, making me upset—to all of the things I had to be thankful for.

I chose to practice gratitude every day. I would say, *Thank you, God, for another day of life. Thank you that I can get out of bed, that I can see, that I can hear, that I can walk and talk, that I'm not in the hospital dying. Thank you for my family who loves me. Thank you that I have a home and a place to sleep, food to eat, and clothes to wear. . . .*

When I shifted my focus to all the good things in my life, I realized how good my life was despite my problems.

Gratitude is counting your blessings and thanking your Heavenly Father for them. This daily practice transforms your attitude, your emotions, and your perspective. So no matter what you're going through, you always have a choice to focus on the good things in your life instead of the bad. This will transform your life and your health. Gratitude is the secret to happiness.

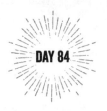

SHINE THROUGH

Courage cannot exist without fear.
    It's what you do when you are afraid that matters.
    Courage is the decision to move forward in spite of fear.
    Fear is the darkness that courage shines through.
    Face your fears. Embrace your fears. Press into them.
    Be strong and courageous today!

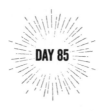

WHEN PEOPLE WRONG YOU . . . REMEMBER THIS

Joseph had 11 brothers and he was his father's favorite. His brothers were so jealous of him that when he was 17 they faked his death and sold him into slavery.[14]

This put Joseph on a completely different path that came with a lot of hardship, but God used it to position him to eventually become the second in command over all of Egypt! His brothers' terrible betrayal set him up for a huge blessing. And years later, he used his power to save his entire family, including his brothers and their families (the nation of Israel), from a seven-year famine. When his brothers bowed down before him, terrified he would put them to death, pleading for mercy, Joseph said to them, "You intended to harm me, but God intended it for good to accomplish what is now being done, the saving of many lives" (Genesis 50:20, NIV).

This radically transformed the way I look at people who wrong me. Instead of letting anger, bitterness, and resentment take over my heart, I choose to quickly forgive them and remind myself that there is a blessing around the corner. So next time someone wrongs you, remember they just set you up for a blessing. The bigger the injury, the bigger the blessing. Expect it. The blessing is coming!

---

14 The story of Joseph's life can be found in Genesis chapters 37–50.

DAY 86

But those who wait on the Lord
Shall renew their strength; They shall
mount up with wings like eagles,
They shall run and not be weary,
They shall walk and not faint.

—Isaiah 40:31 (NKJV)

Don't be impatient. Don't be impulsive. Don't be rash. Don't rush into anything out of fear. Don't do something just for the sake of doing something. Sometimes the best thing to do is nothing. Wait on the Lord. Wait for Him to give you clarity, peace, direction, and confirmation. When you have those things, you can move forward with confidence.

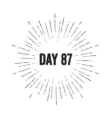

DAY 87

DOUBT IS JUST A THOUGHT, AND YOU CAN CHANGE YOUR THOUGHTS.

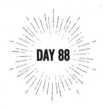

IN THE BELLY OF THE WHALE

Jonah had a calling on his life. God told him to go to Nineveh, but instead he headed in the opposite direction. Then Jonah found himself on a boat in the middle of a violent storm that was threatening to sink the ship.

So Jonah said, "Pick me up and throw me into the sea and it will become calm. I know that it is my fault that this great storm has come upon you" (Jonah 1:12, NIV). They threw him into the sea and the storm subsided. But then a whale swallowed Jonah.

And there he was in the belly of a whale. Jonah could not escape. He was completely powerless. All he could do was sit with his problem. And wait. And pray.

I'm sure Jonah felt hopeless, like this was the end for him. But the whale was taking him somewhere. God used the whale to interrupt Jonah's plans, to get his attention, and to change him. And after three days, the whale spat him out onto dry land, exactly where he was meant to be. And he went to Nineveh.

You may be in the belly of the whale right now, feeling helpless and hopeless. Sit with it. Be still. Listen. And pray. God has a plan for you. And God is using this for your good (Romans 8:28), to change you and to take you to exactly where He wants you to be.

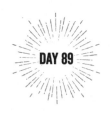

DAY 89

TO ACCOMPLISH GREAT THINGS, WE MUST NOT ONLY ACT, BUT ALSO DREAM; NOT ONLY PLAN, BUT ALSO BELIEVE.

—ANATOLE FRANCE

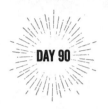

DAY 90

*The most difficult thing is the decision to act,
the rest is merely tenacity.*

—AMELIA EARHART

Tenacity is defined as being able to grip firmly, to hold fast, to hold together, to continue to exist.

Tenacity is your word now. You must embody tenacity.

You must be tenacious.

Do you have a vision and a plan for the future? Grab ahold of it with all of your strength. Flex your mental and spiritual muscles. Hold on tight. Your life depends on it. And don't let go until you get what you want and what you need.

Tenacity pushes through difficult days, disappointment, and discouragement with purpose-driven determination.

You must be persistent. You must be determined. You must to continue to exist.

You are a relentless, unstoppable, tenacious beast!

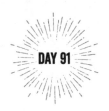

DAY 91

LIFE IS JUST TOO SWEET TO BE BITTER.

—KRIS CARR

Forgiveness turns your bitterness into sweetness.

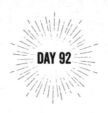

NURTURE, BREATHE, LOVE, AND BELIEVE

Your body is elegant, complex, adaptive, regenerative, and unique. It is an integral and interdependent part of your Being. Your mind, body, soul, and spirit all work together like an orchestra. It is a balance of each of these parts, working together in harmony, that creates a symphony of health.

Nurture
Eat foods that heal. Don't eat foods that harm.

Breathe
Calm your mind and body. Catch those thoughts that create friction or unrest and replace them with thoughts rooted in faith, hope, and gratitude that produce peace and joy.

Love and Support
Choose to love without condition, to love yourself, and to open yourself up to receive support.

Believe
Believe in yourself. Believe that you are worthy of health. Believe in your team. Believe in the medicine that you choose. Believe that cancer is temporary. And above all else, believe that this is part of a much greater purpose and that God will work this for your good.

—THEO HANSON, HUSBAND OF BREAST CANCER SURVIVOR KIM HANSON[15]

15 Connect with Theo and Kim on Instagram @aftercancer.

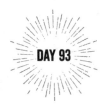

DAY 93

STRENGTH IN WEAKNESS

*And He [God] has said to me, "My grace is sufficient for you,
for power is perfected in weakness." Most gladly, therefore, I
will rather boast about my weaknesses, so that the power of
Christ may dwell in me. Therefore I am well content with
weaknesses, with insults, with distresses, with persecutions,
with difficulties, for Christ's sake; for when I am weak,
then I am strong.*

—2 CORINTHIANS 12:9–10 (NASB)

TRADING PLACES

Some days, when I'm feeling frustrated, discouraged, or unhappy with what's happening around me, when I'm tempted to complain or feel sorry for myself, when things don't go my way, when people treat me badly, when I'm taking all the good things in my life for granted, I have to do a hard reset on my perspective by reminding myself that . . .

> *Right now, there is someone dying in the hospital who would give anything to trade places with you.*

Works every time.

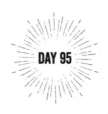

ACTION CREATES MOMENTUM

If you want to go really fast on a bicycle, you've got to pedal. But you can't go from 0 to 10 miles an hour on your first pedal stroke. You go from 0 to 1.

And if you keep pedaling, you will accelerate from 1 to 2, then eventually to 5, then to 10. And if you continue to pedal really hard, you might get up to 15 or even 20 miles an hour. (Now that's fun!) But one pedal push won't get you going fast or get you very far. You have to keep pedaling.

It's harder to move a stationary object than it is to keep a moving object in motion. In physics, this is known as static friction. The hardest part is getting started.

But once you start, your action propels you forward and that produces momentum. From there, continued action maintains or increases your momentum. And just like when you're riding a bike, it's easier to keep up your momentum once you start moving!

So keep moving forward. Keep taking action. Day after day, keep up the intensity. Keep flooding your body with nutrition. Keep exercising. Keep forgiving. Keep choosing to be positive. Keep saying no to temptation and bad habits. Keep reading. Keep researching. Keep trying new things. Keep believing. Keep praying. Keep trusting God.

Keep up the healing momentum!

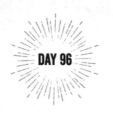

DAY 96

NO MATTER WHAT THE STATISTICS SAY THERE IS ALWAYS A WAY.

—BERNIE SIEGEL

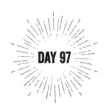

THIS IS YOUR TIME TO HEAL

There is an appointed time for everything.
And there is a time for every event under heaven—
A time to give birth and a time to die;
A time to plant and a time to uproot what is planted.
A time to kill and a time to heal;
A time to tear down and a time to build up.
A time to weep and a time to laugh;
A time to mourn and a time to dance.
A time to throw stones and a time to gather stones;
A time to embrace and a time to shun embracing.
A time to search and a time to give up as lost;
A time to keep and a time to throw away.
A time to tear apart and a time to sew together;
A time to be silent and a time to speak.
A time to love and a time to hate;
A time for war and a time for peace.

—Ecclesiastes 3:1–8 (NASB)

DON'T FEAR FAILURE

Every single piece of technology is the result of millions of failures, from the invention of electricity until now. Millions of tests and failures led to smartphones. There will be mistakes and failures in every endeavor you pursue, including your healing journey. Failing doesn't make you a failure.

Edison famously failed 1,000 times trying to invent the light bulb. It is said that when a reporter asked him, "How did it feel to fail a thousand times?" Edison replied, "I didn't fail a thousand times. The light bulb was an invention with a thousand steps."

Remove your emotion from the equation. When an experiment fails, a scientist says, "Okay, well, now we know that doesn't work. Let's try something else."

Every failure is a discovery. And every failure is a lesson. The fastest way to learn is through mistakes. And failures teach us what doesn't work! Most mistakes and failures aren't actually bad, but even painful and disappointing failures teach powerful and memorable lessons that help you adapt and grow. Failure is necessary; see it as good.

When you fail, don't beat yourself up. Just ask yourself these two questions: *What did I miss? What can I do differently?* And try again.

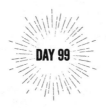

DAY 99

Today I have a question for you inspired by Dr. Lissa Rankin, author of *Mind Over Medicine*:

If you took fear out of the equation, what would that change about how you spend your days?

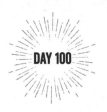

THE LEAP OF FAITH

Faith is trusting God when it is really hard, taking action when you feel paralyzed, moving forward in spite of fear, and stepping out of your comfort zone into the unknown.

There's a scene in *Indiana Jones and the Holy Grail* where Indiana encounters a test called The Leap of Faith. Trying to save his dying father and running out of time, he finds himself facing a deep chasm with no way across. His treasure map has a sketch of a man walking on air across the chasm, so Indiana takes a deep breath and takes a big step off the ledge into thin air, and his foot lands on something. But he appears to be standing on nothing.

Then the camera angle changes, and we see that Indiana Jones is standing on a narrow stone bridge crafted to be an optical illusion, blending in with the rock wall on the other side. The path across the chasm was only invisible from his vantage point at the edge of the cliff.

Some paths are invisible, or seem impossible, and are only illuminated after you take that first scary step.

Don't be afraid to take the first step because you can't see the next one.

Step out in faith into the unknown, and trust your Heavenly Father to reveal your path (Psalm 119:105).

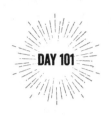

DAY 101

YOU CANNOT SWIM
FOR NEW HORIZONS UNTIL
YOU HAVE THE COURAGE TO
LOSE SIGHT OF THE SHORE.

—ATTRIBUTED TO WILLIAM FAULKNER

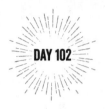

RATHER BE WRONGED

I spent over a decade of my life as a professional real estate investor, property manager, and contractor. And in that time, I was lied to, cheated, and stolen from more than anyone else I know outside that profession.

Imagine how you would feel if you spent your time and money fixing up a house and then the person you rented it to stopped paying rent and refused to move out and trashed the place and you had to hire an attorney and go to court to get them out, costing you thousands of dollars. Now multiply that times 10 or 20 or 50 or hundreds of tenants over the years. Pretty horrifying, right?

Even though I had many wonderful tenants, the negative interactions I was having with bad tenants were turning me into a person who did not like people. I was becoming callous, jaded, cynical, and distrustful. But 1 Corinthians 6:7 changed my outlook. The Apostle Paul says, "Why not rather be wronged? Why not rather be cheated?"

So instead of suing every person who skipped out on rent or tore up my house, I let them wrong me and I forgave them and released them to God. I also learned the most powerful lesson of all: when people wrong you, they set you up for blessing. And now I can actually say thank you to people who've wronged me. And you can too.

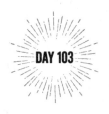

BREAK DOWN

We've all heard the cliché "What doesn't kill you makes you stronger."

When you exercise vigorously, you break down your muscle tissue on purpose so your body will repair and rebuild your muscles stronger than before.

You cannot get stronger without stressing your muscles, pushing them to their limit, and breaking them down.

There are seasons in life where God allows us to go through trials, tribulations, challenges, and difficult circumstances. He does this not to punish us but to stress us and break us down in order to make us stronger—physically, mentally, emotionally, and spiritually.

You may be broken down at the moment, but know that this is only temporary; you will come back stronger.

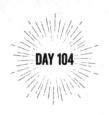

DAY 104

ON MY WORST DAYS UNDERGOING CHEMOTHERAPY FOR LUPUS, I WOULD OBSESSIVELY COUNT MY BLESSINGS UNTIL I WAS CRYING FROM GRATITUDE INSTEAD OF CRYING FROM PAIN.

—BROOKE GOLDNER, M.D.[16]

---

16 Connect with Dr. Brooke Goldner at www.goodbyelupus.com.

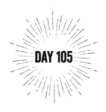

Proverbs 23:7 says that as a man thinks in his heart, so he is.

I find this to be true with all my patients. When a patient believes in their heart that they can overcome cancer, it affects their entire body. Their fight is stronger, their mind is stronger, their body is stronger.

A person doesn't just have breast, ovarian, or colon cancer, because cancer is a disease of the entire body, not just one or two body parts. It isn't just the tumor that needs to be treated; it's all of *you*.

A major part of this process is resolving internal stress and emotional conflict. A roller coaster of thoughts occupies our minds all day to keep us from confronting painful or traumatic events. If left unattended, these internal conflicts will continue to negatively impact your body in many ways, one of which is weakening your immune system.

Daily meditation and positive affirmations can be very helpful in resolving the internal conflicts of your soul.

Cancer has presented you with an opportunity to resolve your internal conflicts, feelings, and past traumas. Now is the time to face what you have buried inside. Emotional healing is the first step to beating cancer. Do not neglect it. Believe you can overcome cancer and live an awesome life!

—*Leigh Erin Connealy, M.D., author of* The Cancer Revolution[17]

---

17 Connect with Dr. Leigh Erin Connealy at www.connealymd.com.

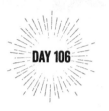

DAY 106

Unexpressed negative emotions never die.
They fester like an infection and become cancerous.

—Chris Voss

Don't bite your tongue and bottle up your negative thoughts, feelings, and emotions. You have to let them out. Don't be afraid of being perceived as impolite or rude, of how others may react, or of someone not liking you.

In *Walden*, Henry David Thoreau famously said, "The mass of men lead lives of quiet desperation."

If you have been leading a life of quiet desperation, now is the time to be noisy. Speak up. Say what you need to say.

If things are happening around you that you don't like, say something. When people frustrate you, tell them. When they upset you, tell them. If you don't like their behavior, tell them. If they are driving you bonkers, tell them. If they are treating you badly, tell them. If you don't want to be around them, tell them.

Express yourself. Free your wildly destructive negative thoughts and emotions before they tear up the cage you've kept them in.

Let them out and let them go.

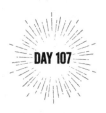

WALKING ON WATER

Peter, seeing Jesus walking on water and full of faith, stepped out of the boat, and began to walk on the water toward Jesus (Matthew 14:29–31).

But he took his eyes off Jesus, and the strong wind and the waves filled him with fear and he began to sink. Then he cried out for help and Jesus rescued him.

You may feel like you are walking on water right now. The big waves around you are scary and threatening to drown you. Fix your eyes on Jesus. He is the author and perfecter of your faith. He has the power to calm the storm, rescue you, lift you out of the waves, and carry you to safety.

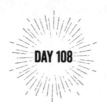

WHO'S DRIVING?

Are you driven by your mind or your emotions?

Your mind is rational. Your emotions are irrational. If you let your emotions drive, your feelings will determine your actions. But your feelings are fickle. They change constantly. And your feelings often become an excuse for not doing what you need to do.

If you only went to work on the days when you felt like going to work, you would miss a lot of workdays and get fired. The reason you show up for work when you don't feel like it is because there are consequences if you don't.

When it comes to our daily choices, including whether or not to take care of ourselves, we tend to let our emotions rule. Our fluctuating feelings, insecurities, fears, and doubts can lead us to self-sabotage through inaction or poor choices. But the consequences are not immediate. They take time to manifest, often as chronic disease.

It's easy to let your emotions drive you, but you don't have to. Your mind controls your actions. And you can choose to resist emotion-driven actions. Like holding your tongue or walking away from an argument. Like choosing to eat an apple when you want to eat ice cream. Like exercising when you really want to lie in bed and binge-watch TV.

Today's Declaration: *I rule my emotions.*

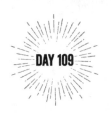

DAY 109

THE LIFE OF YOUR DREAMS IS ON THE OTHER SIDE OF FEAR.

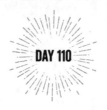

Oh, what joy for those whose disobedience is forgiven, whose sin is put out of sight! Yes, what joy for those whose record the Lord has cleared of guilt, whose lives are lived in complete honesty!

When I refused to confess my sin, my body wasted away, and I groaned all day long. Day and night your heavy hand of discipline was heavy on me. My strength evaporated like water in the summer heat.

Finally, I confessed all my sins to you and stopped trying to hide my guilt. I said to myself, "I will confess my rebellion to the Lord." And you forgave me! All my guilt is gone.

Therefore, let all the godly pray to you while there is still time, that they may not drown in the floodwaters of judgment.

For you are my hiding place; you protect me from trouble. You surround me with songs of victory.

—Psalm 32:1–7 (NLT)

Guilt and shame from sin lead to illness. But confession (admitting your sin) and repentance (turning away from it) lead to freedom and healing. If you are holding on to things in your life that you know are wrong, this is a gentle and loving reminder to surrender them to God. Ask for forgiveness, knowing that your Heavenly Father loves you so much and is ready and willing to forgive you and heal you and welcome you into His loving arms.

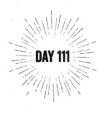

DAY 111

It's no use going back to yesterday,
because I was a different person then.

—LEWIS CARROLL, *ALICE'S ADVENTURES IN WONDERLAND*

Every day changes us. And some days change us a lot. You are a different person now, especially after a cancer diagnosis. And your life should reflect that. Cancer has given you a permission slip to undergo radical life change. Change is good! Embrace this new season of change. Embrace the new you that you are becoming!

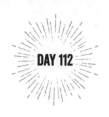

THEN [JESUS] SAID TO THE MAN,
"STRETCH OUT YOUR HAND."
SO HE STRETCHED IT OUT AND IT
WAS COMPLETELY RESTORED,
JUST AS SOUND AS THE OTHER. BUT
THE PHARISEES WENT OUT AND
PLOTTED HOW THEY MIGHT KILL
JESUS. AWARE OF THIS, JESUS
WITHDREW FROM THAT PLACE.
A LARGE CROWD FOLLOWED HIM,
AND HE HEALED ALL WHO WERE ILL.

—MATTHEW 12:13–16 (NIV)

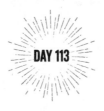

GOLDEN FLAWS

We've been conditioned by culture to believe that beauty is flawless. But flaws can be even more beautiful.

Kintsugi is the ancient Japanese art of repairing broken pottery. But unlike traditional methods of pottery repair, the goal of which is to hide the cracks and damage, kintsugi involves repairing the cracks with gold dust epoxy.

Highlighting and accentuating the cracks with gold celebrates the item's history, making it more beautiful, unique, and precious. Some Japanese artists would even break fine dishes and bowls and repair them with gold on purpose to make them more valuable!

Similarly, *wabi-sabi* is the wonderful Japanese philosophy of seeing beauty in the flawed or imperfect.

Every scar has a story. Maybe it is a lesson learned, a crazy adventure, a story of triumph over adversity, or a story of survival.

Your imperfections, flaws, and scars are beautiful and unique, and they make you more valuable. Don't hide them in shame or embarrassment. Shine a light on them! Show them off!

Decorate your scars in "gold" and use them to tell your unique and amazing story. And instead of criticizing, choose to see the beauty in the flaws and imperfections of others.

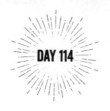

The Lord says, "I will guide you along the best pathway for your life. I will advise you and watch over you.

Do not be like a senseless mule that needs a bit and bridle to keep it under control."

Many sorrows come to the wicked, but unfailing love surrounds those who trust the Lord.

So, rejoice in the Lord and be glad, all you who obey Him! Shout for joy all you whose hearts are pure!

—PSALM 32:8–11 (NLT)

This passage has a wonderful promise and a sober warning. First, the warning. Don't be like a "senseless mule" that doesn't mind, wanders off, and requires constant correction, discipline, and control. If you cannot control yourself—if you pursue sinful and wicked things, or if you indulge in bad or self-destructive behavior—you can expect many troubles and sorrows in life.

But those who trust in the Lord are surrounded by unfailing love! Doesn't that sound like a better option? And isn't it wonderful to know that your Heavenly Father loves you so much that he promises to guide you along the best path for your life, to advise you and to watch over you and protect you?

Trust and obey the Lord. Rejoice and be glad. And shout for joy every once in a while!

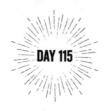

You are the navigator of your journey and the author of your story.

Don't let anyone rush you into things you don't understand.

Don't do anything that doesn't make sense to you.

Don't let anyone take the wheel from you.

Don't let anyone manipulate you with fear.

Make decisions that are based on facts and faith, not fear.

Listen to your instincts and intuition.

Listen to your gut.

Listen to the Holy Spirit.

Pray. Reach out. Ask God for help.

Ask for signs. Ask for direction. Ask God to show you what you need to do and what you need to change.

Both faith and doubt are choices.

Choose faith.

DAY 116

WAIT FOR THE LORD; BE STRONG AND LET YOUR HEART TAKE COURAGE; YES, WAIT FOR THE LORD.

—PSALM 27:14 (NASB)

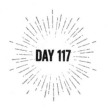

DAY 117

Once the search is in progress, something will be found.

—Brian Eno and Peter Schmidt, *Oblique Strategies*

Sometimes, after you've put in a lot of effort, things you try don't work. And you get frustrated. And you feel stuck, or you feel like you have to start over. And you want to give up.

Don't let disappointment and discouragement paralyze you.

Some answers are easy to find, and some answers take time. Sometimes the easy-to-find answers—common knowledge—turn out to be only half right or completely wrong.

This is a reminder to keep searching.

You have to keep looking. Keep reading. Keep researching. Keep learning. Keep trying new things. Keep talking to people. Keep asking your Heavenly Father for help. Keep asking people for help.

Don't stop. And don't give up.

Keep searching, because if you keep searching . . .

Something will be found!

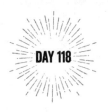

DAY 118

*Praise the Lord, my soul; and forget not all His benefits—
who forgives all your sins and heals all your diseases, who
redeems your life from the pit, and crowns you with love
and compassion, who satisfies your desires with good
things, so that your youth is renewed like the eagle's.*

—Psalm 103:1–5 (NIV)

*Lord, I praise you and I thank you for everything you have done
for me. Thank you for another day of life. Thank you for forgiving me and for healing me. Thank you for saving my life. Thank
you for your love and compassion. Thank you for satisfying the
desires of my heart. Thank you for renewing my strength.*

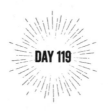

WHO'S RESPONSIBLE?

There are three types of people connected to every problem. Those who caused the problem, those affected, and those who need to solve it.

In a perfect world, those responsible for causing a problem would be willing and able to solve it.

In the real world, people often take responsibility for solving problems they did not cause because those problems have become their problems or because they want to help solve those problems for others.

Sometimes taking responsibility means taking the blame, but at other times it means taking ownership of a problem that you didn't cause.

Regardless of who caused the problem or whose fault it is, if you have a problem, it is your responsibility to solve it.

If you have cancer, you may have multiple problems. . . .

If you solve enough problems, you get well.

Accept responsibility and be a problem solver.

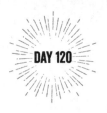

GIVING YOUR FEAR TO GOD

Worry and doubt are the opposite of faith. Exercising your faith means trusting God to lead you, to protect you, to provide for you, and to heal you. Fully trusting Him means letting go of fear—choosing to believe and not to doubt.

Every time I feel worried and afraid, this is the way I pray:

> *Lord, I am not going to be afraid. I am giving you my fear. Jesus, I am laying it at your feet. I trust you with my life, my health, my family, my finances, my future. I trust you. Thank you for leading me in the path of healing, for supplying all my needs, and for working everything out for my good. Amen.*

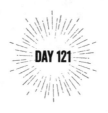

DAY 121

FORGIVENESS RELEASES YOU FROM A PRISON OF PAIN.

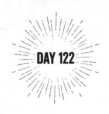

NO ONE'S GONNA DO IT FOR YOU

When our son was diagnosed with stage IV cancer just before his first birthday, we owned the fact that no one cared whether he made it more than we did. And we turned our life upside down to help him survive. Our home became a healing center.

You need to come into total alignment with this truth: Whatever needs to happen, it's on you to ensure that it happens. You have to help yourself heal.

Don't have the money for supplements and treatments? Figure out how to get a donation or a discount. Feel like you can't navigate the waters of healing? Find knowledgeable doctors and coaches to help you. They are out there.

God has gifted us with so many tools to thrive—plants, energies, even our own thoughts! There's never a reason to say, "There's nothing else I can do."

Walk barefoot in the woods. Fundraise. Juice. Ask for discounts. Meditate. Research. Laugh. There's no time to feel down. . . . You've got too much healing to do!

Trust in God, but row away from the rocks.

—*Ryan and Teddy Sternagel*[18]

---

18 Connect with Ryan and Teddy Sternagel at www.thesternmethod.com.

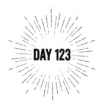

DAY 123

Faith is taking the first step, even when you can't see the whole staircase.

—ATTRIBUTED TO MARTIN LUTHER KING, JR.

I definitely could not see the whole staircase when I took a step of faith to choose nutrition and natural therapies instead of chemotherapy after surgery. The fear of suffering and death was real. But I believed that healing was possible. I believed I could get well. And I mustered up enough faith to take the first step, believing that God was with me and that He would guide me. My faith was proven by my action. And with each step, the fear decreased and my confidence grew. I've ascended a lot of steps in the last 16 years, and the view from up here is fantastic. You have that to look forward to. Don't worry about the whole staircase. Just focus on the next step and take it.

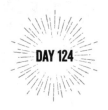

DAY 124

In her books, *Radical Remission* and *Radical Hope*, Kelly Turner, Ph.D., explores the 10 common factors that cancer patients who survive against the odds have in common:

- Having strong reasons for living
- Taking control of your health
- Radically changing your diet
- Exercising
- Using herbs and supplements
- Following your intuition
- Deepening your spiritual connection
- Releasing suppressed emotions
- Increasing positive emotions
- Embracing social support

Notice only three of these factors are physical: diet, supplements, and exercise. The rest are mental, emotional, social, and spiritual.

Based on this, one could make the case that 70 percent of healing is *not* physical. Your physical health is a reflection of your mental, emotional, social, and spiritual health.

Radically changing your diet, exercising, and taking herbs and supplements will be beneficial. But if you are only addressing the physical stuff, you are not doing enough.

Everything must be addressed. Everything must change.

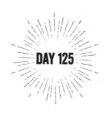

NO PERSON HAS THE POWER TO HAVE EVERYTHING THEY WANT, BUT IT IS IN THEIR POWER NOT TO WANT WHAT THEY DON'T HAVE, AND TO CHEERFULLY PUT TO GOOD USE WHAT THEY DO HAVE.

—UNKNOWN, ATTRIBUTED TO SENECA

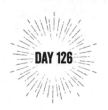

THE FUTURE IS NOW

Your life today is the sum total of all the decisions you've made in the past.

And your future life will be created by the decisions you make now. Today.

Your future is not preprogrammed.

You are not a victim of fate.

Your destiny is determined by you.

Your choices matter.

Your choices today create your future tomorrow.

So make good choices today!

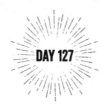

DAY 127

FAITH WITHOUT ACTION IS FANTASY.

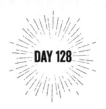

Give me a lever long enough . . . and I shall move the world.

—Archimedes

Every action produces a result. Think of every choice you make and every action you take as levers. You have big levers and small levers.

Big levers produce the biggest results. Big levers are eating a whole-food, plant-based diet rich in fruits and vegetables. Daily exercise. At least eight hours of sleep each night. Quitting smoking, drinking, or using drugs. Reducing your stress. Getting right with God. Repentance and forgiveness. Big levers can also be quitting a job you hate, moving, or ending a toxic relationship.

Small levers have a small benefit or no benefit. Many people make the mistake of pulling small levers (like taking supplements) because they are easy while ignoring the big levers (like changing their diet). And they typically don't get good results.

When faced with any challenge, it's important to prioritize your steps. Ask yourself, *What are the biggest levers I can pull?*

Pull the biggest levers first. And once you've pulled all of the big levers, then move on to the smaller ones.[19]

---

19 Some cancer therapies are big levers with undesirable side effects and long-term consequences. Investigation is required.

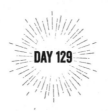

RUN AWAY

Remember how much you loved to run as a kid?
> Go for a run today.
> A short run.
> A long run.
> Some running, some walking.
> Run as much as possible, even if it's only for a few seconds.
> Feel what it's like to run and be alive.
> Movement is life.
> Run, baby, run!

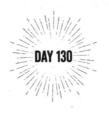

HOWEVER, AS IT IS WRITTEN: "WHAT NO EYE HAS SEEN, WHAT NO EAR HAS HEARD, AND WHAT NO HUMAN MIND HAS CONCEIVED"—THE THINGS GOD HAS PREPARED FOR THOSE WHO LOVE HIM.

—1 CORINTHIANS 2:9 (NIV)

Your Heavenly Father loves you so much and has wonderful, amazing, incredible things in store for you—things too wonderful, amazing, and incredible for you to even imagine. Believe it!

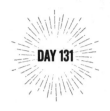

DAY 131

FORGIVENESS IS A COURAGEOUS ACT.

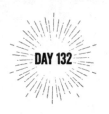

DAY 132

The Lord helps the fallen
and lifts those bent beneath their loads. . . .
He grants the desires of those who fear Him;
he hears their cries for help and rescues them.

—Psalm 145:14,19 (NLT)

Father, thank you that you hear my cries for help, that you will lift
me up, that you will rescue me, and that you will grant my desires.

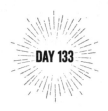

IN THE MIDDLE OF FEAR IS WHEN YOU EXERCISE YOUR FAITH

Fear is a test of your faith. If you're fearful and doubting, then you are not in faith.

You can't doubt and believe at the same time. You have to choose one or the other.

You have the power to choose to believe that God loves you, that He has a plan to prosper you and not to harm you (Jeremiah 29:11), and that He will work everything out for your good (Romans 8:28).

You have the power to choose to trust your Heavenly Father.

You have the power to choose not to be afraid—to give all the "what-ifs," the uncertainty, and the fear of what could be to Him, today and every day.

Exercise your faith in the middle of fear.

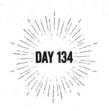

*Because of the Lord's great love we are not consumed,
for his compassions never fail. They are new every
morning; great is your faithfulness.*

*I say to myself, "The Lord is my portion;
therefore I will wait for him."*

*The Lord is good to those whose hope is in him,
to the one who seeks him; it is good to wait
quietly for the salvation of the Lord. . . .*

*I called on your name, Lord, from the depths of the pit.
You heard my plea: "Do not close your ears to my cry for relief."
You came near when I called you, and you said, "Do not fear."
You, Lord, took up my case; you redeemed my life.*

—LAMENTATIONS 3:22–26,55–58 (NIV)

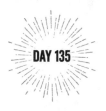

BEWARE

Energy vampires drain your energy. They are selfish, self-centered people. They're narcissistic, inconsiderate, needy, critical, and often play the victim in order to take advantage of you, manipulate you, or abuse you. People like this will suck the life out of you.

You need to get away from energy vampires. If you're in an abusive relationship, get out of there as quickly as possible. Hopefully, you can restore that relationship over time. But for now you need to free yourself. If it's someone you don't live with—like a sibling, friend, or coworker—you should either end the relationship or redefine the terms. If you want to stay close but you don't like the way someone is treating you, you need to be clear about how their actions make you feel and set some new boundaries. For example: "I know you love me, but you need to stop criticizing me. It makes me not want to be around you."

Today's Reflection: *Are there energy vampires in your life that you need to get away from?*

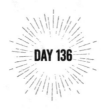

WHO ARE YOU LISTENING TO?

*For God has not given us a spirit of fear, but of power
and of love and of a sound mind.*

—2 Timothy 1:7 (NKJV)

We all listen to lots of people: family, friends, doctor, neighbor, pastor, the news . . . but there's another source of influence that often goes unnoticed. In times of uncertainty, it creeps into our minds. It has the power to overrule our experience, education, and even our God-given instincts. It binds our hands, freezes our thoughts, and deafens our ability to hear from others, including God Himself.

I'm talking about fear. Fear can be a powerful, paralyzing force. But fear has an Achilles' heel: faith.

Faith and fear are both concerned with the future. But faith looks at the uncertainty of tomorrow with confidence, rooted in the grace and mercy of God, and chooses to believe that good things are coming. Faith unlocks love and provides hope for the future. Faith gives strength to face a new day and lights a clear path forward. We have been given a powerful spirit of faith. And it is through faith that we are healed.

Throw off your fear by embracing your spirit of faith. And listen well.

—*Kevin Campbell*[20]

---

20 Kevin's wife, Cortney, was diagnosed with NLP Hodgkin's lymphoma in 2008 and healed with nutrition and nontoxic therapies. Learn more at www.anticancermom.com.

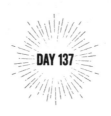

DAY 137

CAST YOUR BURDEN UPON THE LORD AND HE WILL SUSTAIN YOU; HE WILL NEVER ALLOW THE RIGHTEOUS TO BE SHAKEN.

—PSALM 55:22 (NASB)

DON'T EXCUSE YOURSELF

There is no limit to the number of excuses available to a person who does not want to do something.

Excuses prevent you from taking action, paralyze your progress, trap you in victimhood, and keep you from getting better (at everything).

Excuses are always easier than action. And you have an unlimited supply of them.

Excuses feel like legitimate reasons. But they rarely are. Excuses often manifest as busyness: doing things that are less important than the thing you really need to do. Many days, I caught myself making embarrassingly trivial excuses not to sit down and work on this book. And some days I let the excuses win.

Excuses get you nowhere. They keep you frozen in place, like Han Solo in carbonite. Nothing changes, you don't improve, your problems don't go away, and your frustration and unhappiness grow. So you can make excuses or you can make progress. You have the power to make that choice every day.

Today's Reflection: *What excuses are you making for not doing the things you should be doing?*

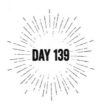

Who of you by worrying can add a single hour to your life?

—Jesus
—Luke 12:25 (NIV)

Worrying does nothing for you. By nothing, I mean nothing good for you. Worrying will not extend your life. It will shorten it. And it will make you stressed, fearful, and miserable in the meantime. Who wants that? Worrying is a pointless waste of energy and emotion. It will not help you, and it will definitely hurt you. Worries are toxic thoughts, and worrying is a bad habit that steals your joy and weakens your immune system. When you worry, you are actively not trusting your Heavenly Father to supply all of your needs. Don't do it.

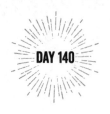

DAY 140

THOUGHTS ARE CHEMICAL. THEY CAN EITHER KILL US OR CURE US.

—BERNIE SIEGEL

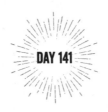

ACCORDING TO YOUR FAITH

*As Jesus went on from there, two blind men followed
Him, crying out, "Have mercy on us, Son of David!"*

*When He entered the house, the blind men came up to Him, and
Jesus said to them, "Do you believe that I am able to do this?"*

They said to Him, "Yes, Lord."

*Then He touched their eyes, saying, "It shall be done to
you according to your faith." And their eyes were opened.*

—Matthew 9:27–29 (NASB)

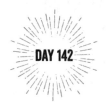

DAY 142

Go to bed a little smarter each day.

—Warren Buffett

You can't get smart in one day. You can't become an expert in one day. You can't learn everything you need to know in one day. You can't solve all your problems in one day. You can't get healthy in one day.

But each day, if you make time to read and research, to educate yourself, to learn new things, you will increase your knowledge. And day by day, you will get a little smarter. And that's like earning compound interest on your intelligence.

To increase your retention, journal or take notes on what you learn each day. It might even turn into a book someday. . . .

It's important to focus on learning new things that are most useful to you. For example, I'm sure watching a documentary on African elephants would be fascinating and filled with lots of interesting facts, but none of them would be useful to help you get healthy.

This incremental daily improvement strategy also applies to healthy eating, exercise, and your spiritual life.

The small disciplines you practice each day add up to big results over time. Go to bed a little smarter today.

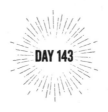

THE REWARDS OF WISDOM

How blessed is the man who finds wisdom and the man who gains understanding. For her profit is better than the profit of silver and her gain better than fine gold. She is more precious than jewels; and nothing you desire compares with her. Long life is in her right hand; in her left hand are riches and honor. Her ways are pleasant ways and all her paths are peace.

—Proverbs 3:13–17 (NASB)

Blessings. A long life. Riches. Honor. Peace. That's what you want, right? Make gaining wisdom and understanding a primary pursuit. Wisdom and understanding come from a desire to learn, followed by thorough research. Set aside your preconceived notions. Humble yourself. Accept that what you think you know may be wrong. And keep reading, keep researching, keep learning, and keep growing. Wisdom and understanding and all of their rewards are coming!

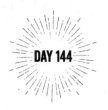

DAY 144

*He who jumps into the void owes no explanation
to those who stand and watch.*

—Jean-Luc Godard

You've taken a leap of faith into the unknown, into the void.
You are taking massive, radical life-changing action to survive and thrive. You are becoming a different person. Your
friends and family are scratching their heads. They think
you've lost your mind. . . . It's okay. Don't worry about what
they think of you. They don't understand what it's like to be
in survival mode. You don't have to explain yourself. They
will understand eventually.

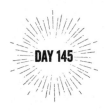

MAKE AMENDS

If there are people in your life with whom you are out of sorts, you need to make amends. That means asking for forgiveness from the people you've hurt.

I suggest you say something like this:

"This cancer diagnosis has made me realize what's important, and I just want you to know that I'm really, really sorry about [that thing you did]. I was wrong, and I hope you'll forgive me."

The best-case scenario is that the person says, "I'm sorry too. I forgive you. I love you. Let's hug." But they may say, "I don't care. I hate you and I'll never forgive you," and other harsh things. If that happens, don't make excuses, don't defend yourself, and don't retaliate. Just let them say what they need to say and respond with "I understand why you feel the way you do, and I just want you to know that I really am sorry."

Humble yourself, admit you were wrong, and ask for forgiveness. This is the most important first step to mending a broken relationship. They may not forgive you right away, or ever. And that's okay. But the weight of guilt and shame will be lifted off you after you ask for forgiveness. And then you can move forward.

Today's Challenge: *Who do you need to make amends with?*

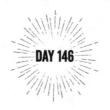

LAUGH IT UP!

Some of the best things in life are free. And it just so happens that one of the best immune-boosting, health-promoting practices you can incorporate into your life is also free. It's laughter.

Laughter is powerful medicine! Laughter releases endorphins in your brain, increases blood flow and oxygenation in your body, improves your mood, reduces stress hormones, relieves pain, and even boosts your immune system. One study found that people who watched an hour of stand-up comedy had increased activity of their natural killer cells, B-cells, T-cells, and immunoglobulins.[21] And some of these anti-cancer immune-boosting effects lasted for up to 12 hours!

---

21 Berk et al., "Modulation of Neuroimmune Parameters During the Eustress of Humor-Associated Mirthful Laughter," *Alternative Therapies in Health and Medicine* 7, no. 2 (March 2001): 62–72, 74–76. https://www.ncbi.nlm.nih.gov/pubmed/11253418.

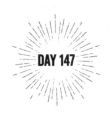

DAY 147

DO NOT FEAR, FOR I AM WITH YOU;
DO NOT ANXIOUSLY LOOK ABOUT
YOU, FOR I AM YOUR GOD. I WILL
STRENGTHEN YOU, SURELY I WILL
HELP YOU, SURELY I WILL UPHOLD
YOU WITH MY RIGHTEOUS
RIGHT HAND.

—ISAIAH 41:10 (NASB)

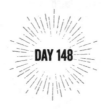

ASK FOR HELP

Do you feel helpless? Ask for help.

If you've ever helped someone in need, then you know it is a joy and privilege to help others. People want to help you!

Help is ready and waiting for you to ask.

Don't try to do everything yourself. You can't.

Asking for help is a courageous act of humility because in doing so you show your weakness and vulnerability.

A prideful person never asks for help. Don't let pride get in the way of getting the help you need.

And don't get upset with the people around you for not helping if you haven't told them what you need. No one can read your mind.

Be specific. Get clear on your needs. Make a list. Humble yourself and ask for help.

Ask and you shall receive (Matthew 7:7)!

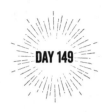

DAY 149

In fact, this is love for God: to keep his commands. And his commands are not burdensome, for everyone born of God overcomes the world. This is the victory that has overcome the world, even our faith. Who is it that overcomes the world? Only the one who believes that Jesus is the Son of God. . . .

This is the confidence we have in approaching God: that if we ask anything according to his will, he hears us. And if we know that he hears us—whatever we ask— we know that we have what we asked of him.

—1 John 5:3–5,14–15 (NIV)

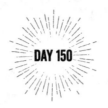

DAY 150

A wise man is strong, and a man of knowledge increases power. For by wise guidance you will wage war, and in abundance of counselors there is victory.

—PROVERBS 24:5–6 (NASB)

You need counselors. Get a second opinion, and a third, and a fourth. Take the time to ask for help and guidance from people you know and trust. Assemble a mastermind group, a brain trust, or a "board of directors" of friends, family, doctors, and wellness professionals to help increase your wisdom and knowledge to guide you in your healing journey. In the abundance of counselors there is victory!

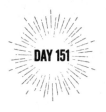

Surely the righteous will never be shaken;
they will be remembered forever.
They will have no fear of bad news;
their hearts are steadfast, trusting in the Lord.

—Psalm 112:6–7 (NIV)

Trust the Lord with all your heart. Do not fear bad news. You will not be shaken by it!

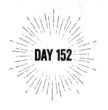

DAY 152

The more you do, the more you fail. The more you fail, the more you learn. The more you learn, the better you get.

—John C. Maxwell

The first day I tried to snowboard, I failed (ahem, fell) over and over. I fell on my butt. I fell on my face. I fell getting *on* the lift. I fell getting *off* the lift. I skidded, flipped, and rolled down the mountain all day. It was frustrating, painful, and comical. By the end of the day, my clothes were caked in ice and snow from head to toe. Every muscle was sore. And my body was one big bruise. Day two wasn't much better. But on day three I had a breakthrough. I wasn't falling down as much. I was starting to get it! All that failure was making me better. I persevered through countless failures over multiple trips and I learned how to snowboard. Failure is necessary and good and an essential part of life and growth. Don't fear failure. Failure is the best teacher. Do. Fail. Learn. Grow.

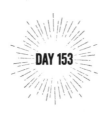

DAY 153

COURAGE DOESN'T ALWAYS ROAR. SOMETIMES COURAGE IS THE QUIET VOICE AT THE END OF THE DAY WHISPERING, "I WILL TRY AGAIN TOMORROW."

—MARY ANNE RADMACHER

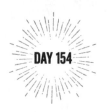

YOUR TRUE CHARACTER IS REVEALED IN ADVERSITY

It is easy to be happy and hopeful when everything is going well. But it takes faith and a healthy measure of character to walk through "the valley of the shadow of death."

Your character is not just who you are; it is how you are. It guides you in actions, decisions, and mental well-being. Your character determines how you experience this moment, at this time—both internally and externally.

You are being refined like precious metal. You are being made ready for a purpose that is something bigger, something more beautiful than you can imagine. Your character is being challenged to be courageous, compassionate, decisive, patient, faithful, and grateful. You are being challenged to break free from fear and to live an abundant life in the midst of difficulty.

Do not let fear or suffering cause you to waver from your convictions to heal and to thrive. Instead, remain steadfast with the peace and knowledge that this adversity is temporary and the character you develop is eternal.

—*Theo Hanson*[22]

---

22 Theo's wife, Kim, was diagnosed with breast cancer in 2014 and healed with nutrition and non-toxic therapies. Connect with them at www.thevidaprotocol.com.

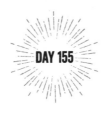

"FOR I KNOW THE PLANS
I HAVE FOR YOU," DECLARES
THE LORD, "PLANS TO PROSPER
YOU AND NOT TO HARM YOU, PLANS
TO GIVE YOU HOPE AND A FUTURE."

—JEREMIAH 29:11 (NIV)

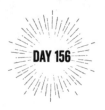

FIGHT THE RESISTANCE

Most of us have two lives. The life we live and the unlived life within us. Between the two stands resistance.

Any act that rejects immediate gratification in favor of long-term growth, health, or integrity. Or, expressed in another way, any act that derives from our higher nature instead of our lower. Any of these will elicit resistance.[23]

—STEVEN PRESSFIELD

Resistance is fueled by fear and self-doubt. Resistance is the force inside you that doesn't want to eat healthy or exercise or forgive. Resistance doesn't "feel like it." Resistance doesn't want you to change, or heal, or do the most important things you know you must do to transform your life. Resistance leads to excuses.

Resistance is your enemy. And you must fight the resistance.

Giving in to resistance makes you feel worse. But every time you push through and overcome resistance, you feel better. And you get better at it. You get stronger and smarter and more confident. Some days are easier than others, but the most important thing is to recognize resistance when you feel it. And then you can make a conscious decision to fight and overcome it.

---

23 Quotes from and interpretation inspired by *The War of Art* by Steven Pressfield.

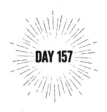

Blessed is he who considers the poor;
The Lord will deliver him in time of trouble.
The Lord will preserve him and keep him alive,
And he will be blessed on the earth;
You will not deliver him to the will of his enemies.
The Lord will strengthen him on his bed of illness;
You will sustain him on his sickbed.

—PSALM 41:1–3 (NKJV)

Do you want to be delivered from trouble? Do you want to be blessed? Do you want to be kept alive, strengthened, and sustained through illness? These are the rewards for those who care for the needs of the poor.

Today's Challenge: *Look for opportunities to give to those in need. Find a charity to support financially or to donate your time to. Prepare to give in advance. Keep cash in your wallet for that purpose, and when the opportunity arises, you will be ready, willing, and able!*

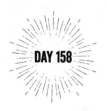

DAY 158

But those who wait on the Lord
Shall renew their strength;
They shall mount up with wings like eagles,
They shall run and not be weary,
They shall walk and not faint.

—Isaiah 40:31 (NKJV)

I love this verse so much. What a beautiful promise. Can you picture yourself soaring and running? I bet you can't wait!

But waiting is hard. We want immediate answers and everything fixed, like, yesterday.

Our timing is impatient, rushed, and flawed. And we often rush into things that promise a quick fix but that ultimately aren't beneficial and can even delay our progress. Because we want results *now*. But God's timing is perfect.

Waiting on the Lord means slowing down. Pressing pause. Taking a step back and asking God, "Okay. What are you trying to show me? What in my life do I need to change?"

And then, wait for direction. If you don't have direction . . . if you don't have peace about your next steps, you don't have to take them. You can wait.

Wait until you have the answer you need, clear direction, and peace.

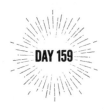

BY HIS WOUNDS

*For you have been called for this purpose, since Christ also
suffered for you, leaving you an example for you to follow in
His steps, who committed no sin, nor was any deceit found in His
mouth; and while being reviled, He did not revile in return; while
suffering, He uttered no threats, but kept entrusting* Himself
*to Him who judges righteously; and He Himself bore our sins in
His body on the cross, so that we might die to sin and live to
righteousness; for by His wounds you were healed.*

—1 Peter 2:21–24 (NASB)

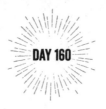

DAY 160

PRESS ON

Nothing in the world can take the place of persistence. Talent will not; nothing is more common than unsuccessful men with talent. Genius will not; unrewarded genius is almost a proverb. Education will not; the world is full of educated derelicts. Persistence and determination are omnipotent. The slogan "Press on" has solved and always will solve the problems of the human race.

—CALVIN COOLIDGE

There are ups and downs in the healing journey. Successes and disappointments. Advances and setbacks. Through it all, be persistent and tenacious. Persistence overcomes obstacles. Tenacity doesn't let go. Determination never gives up. Press on!

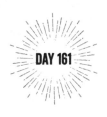

NO MATTER HOW MUCH GOOD YOU DO,
THERE WILL ALWAYS BE SOMEONE WHO
THINKS YOU AREN'T DOING IT RIGHT,
YOU AREN'T DOING ENOUGH, OR YOU ARE
DOING IT FOR THE WRONG REASONS.
DON'T WORRY ABOUT THE CRITICS.

JUST KEEP DOING GOOD!

DAY 162

And we know that in all things God works for the good of those who love him, who have been called according to His purpose.

—Romans 8:28 (NIV)

Notice that this is a conditional promise for those who love God. So what does it mean to love God?

Jesus said, "I am the way and the truth and the life. No one comes to the Father except through me." He also said, "If you love me, keep my commands" (John 14:6,15, NIV).

Jesus gave a lot of instruction on how to live a life that is pleasing to God. And when He was asked "What is the greatest commandment?" this was his answer:

> *The most important commandment is this: "Listen, O Israel! The Lord our God is the one and only Lord. And you must love the Lord your God with all your heart, all your soul, all your mind, and all your strength." The second is equally important: "Love your neighbor as yourself." No other commandment is greater than these.*
> —Mark 12:29–31 (NLT)

Love God by honoring and obeying Him. And love people through service, treating them the way you would want to be treated. That's how you stay in the blessing and can confidently expect God to work all things for your good!

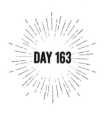

IT DOESN'T NEED TO BE PERFECT. IT JUST NEEDS TO BE.

Don't let inexperience, insecurity, self-doubt, or the need for perfectionism paralyze you and prevent you from taking action . . . from taking care of yourself . . . from pursuing the desires of your heart . . . from fulfilling your purpose . . . from completing your mission . . . from creating the life you have dreamed about.

Perfection should never be the goal. You will never be perfect this side of Heaven.

The goal is continuous improvement.

Healing is a process. And the process involves taking *inspired imperfect action,* without all the knowledge, without all the steps, without all the tools, without a guarantee, but with an understanding that your Heavenly Father will supply all of your needs and with the belief that after each step you will receive what you need to take the next one.

Your plan, your routine, and your protocol do not need to be perfect; they just need to be.

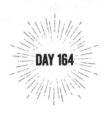

DAY 164

*GREAT CROWDS CAME TO HIM [JESUS],
BRINGING WITH THEM THE LAME,
THE BLIND, THE CRIPPLED, THE MUTE
AND MANY OTHERS, AND LAID THEM
AT HIS FEET; AND HE HEALED THEM.*

—MATTHEW 15:30 (NIV)

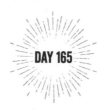

THERE'S SOMEONE YOU NEED TO FORGIVE TODAY

How did I know that? Am I a wizard? No, I am not. I know there is someone you need to forgive because we all have people in our life whom we need to forgive. Nearly every day people hurt us in small ways, and sometimes in enormously painful ways.

You may have multiple people in your life toward whom you've been holding resentment and bitterness. You may have a battalion of offenders in your past. They all need to be forgiven. If you are feeling overwhelmed by the prospect of forgiving them all, and you don't know where to start, here's my advice.

Just pick one person, the person who popped into your mind first, and forgive them today.

Remember: forgiveness is not a feeling. It is a choice. And once you choose to forgive, God will heal your heart. And then your feelings toward that person will change.

Forgive one person today. Give them to God. Surrender your bitterness and anger, and let Him deal with them.

God, I forgive them for _____. I am letting this go. They are all yours. I am asking you to bless them. And forgive me for carrying this bitterness and anger for so long. Thank you for forgiving me. In Jesus's name, Amen.

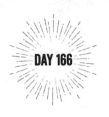

DAY 166

PLEASANT WORDS ARE A HONEYCOMB, SWEET TO THE SOUL AND HEALING TO THE BONES.

—PROVERBS 16:24 (NASB)

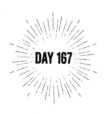

DAY 167

A therapeutic formula to be said repeatedly each morning and evening from French psychologist Émile Coué:

"Every day, in every way, I am getting better and better."

"Every day, in every way, I am getting better and better."

"Every day, in every way, I am getting better and better."

"Every day, in every way, I am getting better and better."

"Every day, in every way, I am getting better and better."

"Every day, in every way, I am getting better and better."

"Every day, in every way, I am getting better and better."

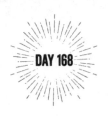

DAY 168

THE WORDS OF THE RECKLESS PIERCE LIKE SWORDS, BUT THE TONGUE OF THE WISE BRINGS HEALING.

—PROVERBS 12:18 (NIV)

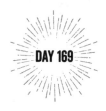

TURN THE TABLES ON "I CAN'T"

If you think you can't do something, you set yourself up for failure.

Because you either don't try or you give up too soon.

Instead of telling yourself you can't do something, which shuts down all possibility of success, ask yourself how you can.

When you are faced with a problem and you find yourself tempted to think or say, "I can't do this," take a step back and ask yourself, "How can I do this?"

This fires up your solution engine, the powerful, creative, problem-solving part of your brain. That's where all of your best ideas come from!

You are smart. You can do so much more that you realize. Believe in yourself. And believe that you can do all things through Christ who gives you strength (Philippians 4:13).

Be creative. Be resourceful. Be a problem solver.

Another powerful thought to replace "I can't" is "I can do this. I just need to figure out how."

Believe you can!

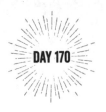

DAY 170

WITHOUT FAITH IT IS IMPOSSIBLE TO PLEASE GOD.

—HEBREWS 11:6 (NIV)

Faith is not complicated. It is simply choosing to believe.

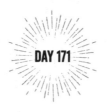

What is a rebel? A man who says no.

—ALBERT CAMUS, *L'HOMME REVOLTÉ*

You are officially a member of the rebellion. Cue the *Star Wars* theme song!

Be a rebel and say no to your bad habits. Say no to junk food. Say no to negative thinking. Say no to laziness. Say no to excuses. Say no to bitterness. Say no to anyone who tries to use or abuse you. Say no to pressure and intimidation and to anything you don't understand. And say yes to anything that promotes life, health, happiness, and healing!

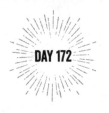

GROWING UP

You are growing and changing.

Not everyone is going to grow and change with you.

Some will even oppose you and resent you for growing.

Don't let them slow you down.

One day some of them will understand and begin growing too.

Others never will.

Decide to be okay with it.

Today's Reflection: *Think about the people in your life whom you are outgrowing. Acknowledge this reality. Take a deep breath. Accept it. Exhale. And release them to be who they are.*

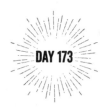

OBSTACLES HAVE A PURPOSE

Obstacles come into your life for one of two reasons: to be overcome or to divert you onto a new path.

Obstacles are meant to challenge you, to push you, to test you, maybe to force you to lighten your load. The more difficult they are, the stronger and wiser you will be when you finally overcome them. Small obstacles are necessary; they prepare you for bigger ones.

Some obstacles, however, cannot be overcome. They are too big. Impassible. Impossible. They force you to take a new path, a "road less traveled." And you may find in hindsight, as I have, that the obstacle that forced you to change direction was a blessing in disguise because you were going the wrong way.

Cancer diverted me onto a new path, forced me to change who I was, and took me to a place and a life that were far better than I could have ever imagined. This is why so many cancer survivors call cancer a blessing or gift.

You can sit defeated at the bottom of an obstacle, wallowing in self-pity, or you can decide to figure out a way over or around it.

Obstacles have a purpose!

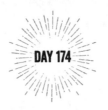

YOUR FAITH HAS MADE YOU . . .

A woman who had had a hemorrhage for 12 years, and had endured much at the hands of many physicians, and had spent all that she had and was not helped at all, but rather had grown worse—after hearing about Jesus, she came up in the crowd behind Him and touched His cloak.

For she thought, "If I just touch His garments, I will get well."

Immediately the flow of her blood was dried up; and she felt in her body that she was healed of her affliction.

Immediately Jesus, perceiving in Himself that the power proceeding from Him had gone forth, turned around in the crowd and said, "Who touched My garments?"

And His disciples said to Him, "You see the crowd pressing in on You, and You say, 'Who touched Me?'" And He looked around to see the woman who had done this.

But the woman fearing and trembling, aware of what had happened to her, came and fell down before Him and told Him the whole truth.

And He said to her, "Daughter, your faith has made you well; go in peace and be healed of your affliction."

—Mark 5:25–34 (NASB)

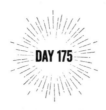

If you are struggling in a particular area, the enemy will keep pressing that issue. Resist him and he will flee!

Keep going, stay positive, and focus on what you are grateful for. Remember: there is always so much to be grateful for, even if bad things are happening too.

This will pass. You will feel good again. Just keep moving forward.

Some days are dark, and so we must go through them. Other days are full of joy and surprises, so let's absorb those days for all that we can, and as much as we can. No matter what the day presents, you can focus on all the things that you have to be grateful for instead of looking at the bad things. There is always something to celebrate.

Remember that there are always more positive things happening at once than negative things. And it could always be worse. So appreciate the now for what it is.

Be here fully.

Don't fight what you can't control. Just surrender and give your heart to God. We overcome evil with good (Romans 12:21)!

—*Liana Werner-Gray, author of* The Earth Diet *and* Cancer Free with Food[24]

24 Connect with Liana Werner-Gray at www.theearthdiet.com.

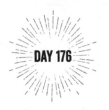

DAY 176

If you can't fly, run. If you can't run, walk. If you can't walk, crawl. But by all means, keep moving.

—Dr. Martin Luther King, Jr.

Some days everything goes smoothly, exactly as planned. You are making tremendous progress. And you are full of faith, hope, and optimism. You are gliding in the wind.

But other days you're grounded. You're down in the mud. The gears are grinding. Your tires are spinning. And you feel like you can't get any traction. It's discouraging. The difficult days are the only ones that make you stronger. And they help you appreciate the easy ones.

Don't let your limitations become excuses for inaction. Do what you *can* do. Some days if all you can do is crawl, then crawl. Just keep moving forward!

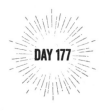

INTO THE WOODS

Studies have shown that *forest bathing*—a fancy term for spending a few hours in the woods—increases natural killer cell activity and reduces blood pressure and stress hormones.[25] Some of these benefits are thought to be from the aromatic compounds, called phytoncides, that are released into the air by trees and plants, which you inhale when you are in the woods.

Being in nature calms you down and boosts your immune system.

Daily exercise is essential to health and healing, and you can compound the benefits of aerobic exercise like walking, running, and dancing by doing it in the woods.

P.S. Don't forget to check for ticks when your forest bath is over.

Today's Challenge: *Schedule time this week to bathe in the forest for a couple hours.*

---

25 Alice Walton, "'Forest Bathing' Really May Be Good for Health, Study Finds," *Forbes*, July 10, 2018. https://www.forbes.com/sites/alicegwalton/2018/07/10/forest-bathing-really-may-be-good-for-health-study-finds/#1fb7452d508e.

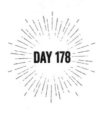

PLAYING THE CANCER CARD

There are good ways to play your cancer card and there are bad ways to play it. If you have cancer and you need help, ask for it! Tell your friends and family what you need. People want to help you, to serve you, and to bless you. Let them.

However, playing your cancer card in order to gain constant attention, sympathy, and pity and to manipulate people into waiting on you hand and foot is a bad strategy. If you use your cancer card to take advantage of people, those people will get tired of you, resent you, and avoid you.

The best way to play your cancer card is to use it to get the help you really need, to relieve yourself from excess obligations, to simplify your life, to get away from people who are not good for you, to reduce your workload, to buy yourself time and freedom, and to reduce your stress.

Use your cancer card sparingly and strategically. Having said all that, if you can use your cancer card to skip the lines at Disney World, by all means, go for it!

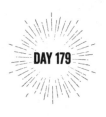

DAY 179

NOTHING IN LIFE IS TO BE FEARED, IT IS ONLY TO BE UNDERSTOOD. NOW IS THE TIME TO UNDERSTAND MORE, SO THAT WE MAY FEAR LESS.

—MARIE CURIE

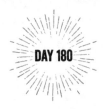

ONE. THING.

One very special day during my surgical residency, I performed my first liver resection all on my own. A critical moment called the Pringle maneuver comes after clamping off blood flow to the entire liver while cutting across the organ. You have to be swift and flawless, because otherwise, spectacularly bad things can happen. . . . When the moment arrived, I confidently requested, "Clamp?" A clamp smacked firmly into my hand. Then the attending surgeon assisting me said, "Hey!" His narrowed eyes peered sternly into mine.

"You're doing one thing right now," he barked. "One. Thing. Do it right."

Those words from Dr. John A. Ryan Jr. struck my core. They color everything I do. Who among us hasn't proudly multitasked throughout the day? But then no single task receives your full-focused best. Sit-ups? Crunch. Feel the burn. Chemo? Bring it. Kill rogue cells. Writing? Inspire. Make words matter. "Mom?" Listen. Put down the phone, match eye levels, say "Yes, honey?" All attention on your child.

Why do it wrong when you can do it right?

Whatever you do—love, learn, eat, fast, pray, meditate, sleep, exercise, give, forgive, believe—"whatever you do, work heartily, as for the Lord and not for men" (Colossians 3:23, ESV).

—*Kristi Funk, M.D.*[26]

---

26 Kristi Funk, M.D., is a breast cancer surgeon, best-selling author, international keynote speaker, and women's health advocate. Connect with her at pinklotus.com/powerup.

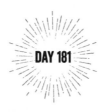

IS CANCER A GIFT?

Many cancer patients refer to cancer as a gift or a blessing, while other patients cringe at that sentiment. I'm kind of in the middle. When I think about gifts or blessings, I think about getting things I actually want, not a life-threatening disease. I love how my friend Kris Carr puts it: "Cancer is not a gift. It's not a pony."

I didn't view cancer as a gift either. Cancer was the worst thing that had ever happened to me. But God worked that terrible thing out for my good. He used it to bless me.

Cancer changed me. It reset my perspective. It humbled me. It made me into a better person. It gave me gratitude for life and health and my loved ones. And it taught me to be content with what I have at every stage of life. Cancer gave me the opportunity to help and encourage others. And today my life is richer and more fulfilled as a result.

Bad things happen in life. The most important thing is that you look for the blessings that come from adversity. It may be hard to imagine, and it may take a little while, but good things will come from the bad because God works all things for the good of those who love Him (Romans 8:28). Blessings are coming. Believe it. And expect them. If you aren't looking for the blessings, you might miss them!

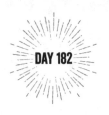

DAY 182

THE PERSON YOU WANT TO FORGIVE LEAST IS THE PERSON YOU NEED TO FORGIVE MOST.

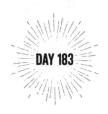

DAY 183

I will lift up my eyes to the mountains;
From where shall my help come?
My help comes from the Lord,
who made heaven and earth.
He will not allow your foot to slip;
He who keeps you will not slumber.
Behold, He who keeps Israel
Will neither slumber nor sleep.
The Lord is your keeper;
The Lord is your shade on your right hand.
The sun will not smite you by day,
nor the moon by night.
The Lord will protect you from all evil;
He will keep your soul.
The Lord will guard your going out and your coming in
From this time forth and forever.

—Psalm 121 (NASB)

DAY 184

I'm not afraid of storms, for I'm learning how to sail my ship.

—Louisa May Alcott, *Little Women*

Wisdom, knowledge, and expertise all come through difficult challenges. The cancer storm is teaching you how to become an expert navigator of life. It is showing you how to live with intention, meaning, and purpose, and how to focus on the essential, how to lighten your load and throw the useless junk overboard, and how to fully trust your Heavenly Father in a way that you never have before. The storm may be difficult, but don't be afraid. You have divine support! Look forward to your life on the other side, when the storm has passed. This storm is teaching you how to sail!

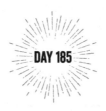

DAY 185

SOME PEOPLE DON'T WANT YOUR HELP. THEY ONLY WANT YOUR ATTENTION.

People who want your help will accept your advice and take action to help themselves. People who only want your attention won't. They will only take advantage of your time and sympathy.

Investing your time and emotional energy to help someone who will not even take the smallest steps to change will only produce worry, frustration, and stress for you.

If a person constantly seeks your advice but does not take action, they really just want your attention. The quicker you can identify this pattern, the less frustration you will feel when they don't take your advice. And the less time and energy you will waste in trying to help them.

Stop wasting your time and energy on people who don't really want your help. And focus on those who do. Serving them will bring you joy and fulfillment.

An alternate strategy for the attention seekers is to give them time and attention, understanding they probably won't take your advice and may never change. This frees you from any emotional responsibility you may be feeling to help them or save them. Now, let's get personal. . . . Are you seeking help from others or just attention?

DAY 186

HEAL ME, LORD, AND I WILL BE HEALED; SAVE ME AND I WILL BE SAVED, FOR YOU ARE THE ONE I PRAISE.

—JEREMIAH 17:14 (NIV)

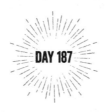

PRACTICE MINDFUL EATING

Food is fuel. Food is life. Food is healing. Food brings pleasure and joy. Food is a gift.

Love your food. Don't just inhale it like a farm animal. Eat without distraction.

Put your phone away. Turn off the TV. Share your meals with loved ones. Or eat in calm solitude. Remind yourself that millions of people around the world go hungry each day and thank your Heavenly Father that you have food to eat. Ask Him to bless it to nourish your body.

Enjoy your food.

Don't rush it. Breathe in the aroma of your meal. Taste every bite. Feel the texture with your tongue as you crush it with your teeth. Chew each bite completely (30-plus times) before swallowing. The better you chew, the more you absorb.

As you eat, remind yourself that you are building a new body. The nutrients in your food will travel to all of your cells and become a part of you.

Food is a blessing. Welcome it into your body with gratitude.

THE WILDERNESS HAS A PURPOSE

God didn't rescue the Israelites from slavery in Egypt to take them into the desert to die. His intention was to take them to a better place, the Promised Land. But they had to cross the wilderness to get there.

During the journey, the Israelites grumbled and complained, doubted, and disobeyed God. They wanted to go back to their life of slavery in Egypt. So God delayed his promise and let them wander in circles in the desert until the entire unbelieving generation of adults had died off. A journey that should have only taken about 11 days on foot lasted 40 years because of their bad attitudes, bad behavior, and unbelief![27]

You may feel like you are in the wilderness right now, wondering why God brought you here. The purpose of the wilderness is to teach you to trust your Heavenly Father completely, to change you, to toughen you up, to prepare you for a new season of life that is better than you can imagine.

Unbelief can delay God's promises in your life and keep you wandering in circles. So exercise your faith and choose to believe that God is leading you through the wilderness and into the Promised Land. Surrender, don't complain, maintain a heart of gratitude, obey, and trust Him completely today.

---

27 You'll find this story in the books Exodus and Numbers.

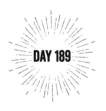

KEEP GOING

Two weeks after radiotherapy it was already back. A lump under my chin tested positive for melanoma, and a CT scan showed the cancer had spread to my neck, lung, and spine.

I felt like a mole in Whac-A-Mole, whacked back into a hole even though I had done everything my doctors recommended. They told me the cancer wouldn't come back, but it had, again and again, and I was devastated, discouraged, and tired of fighting.

My mom gave me a magnet with a quote often attributed to Winston Churchill: "If you're going through hell, keep going." I was going through hell. I wanted to give up, but I knew I had to keep going. And I had to do something different.

By the incredible mercy and grace of God, two and a half months later after changing my treatment approach and beginning to pray faithfully, I was declared free of cancer.

1 Chronicles 28:20 (NASB) says "Be strong and courageous, and act; do not fear nor be dismayed, for the Lord God, my God, is with you. He will not fail you nor forsake you until all the work . . . is finished."

No matter what you've been through or what you're facing, you can be strong and courageous. And you can act. You can take action. I believe in you, and I'm here for you. Trust God and pray. He will finish the good work He started in you!

—*Bailey O'Brien*[28]

---

28 Bailey O'Brien was diagnosed with stage IV melanoma and healed with nutrition and integrative therapies. Connect with her at www.baileyobrien.com.

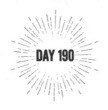

MAKE PLANS FOR THE FUTURE

Document your cancer journey. Journal. Do a video diary. Start a blog. Document what you're doing and what you are learning because when you get well, you can use what you are learning now to help other people.

You need life goals and a clearly defined future to work toward. Making plans for the future is essential to survival.

The spirit-mind-body connection is powerful. When you plan for the future, you are planning to live. You are sending signals of life and health to your subconscious mind and to your body.

Well, I don't know if I'll be here in a year or two years. . . .

Don't be afraid to make plans for the future.

Plan out your life, for the next year, five years, ten years, and beyond. Write down your dreams and your goals. Maybe it's to have kids, or to see your kids graduate college or get married, or to watch your grandchildren grow up, or to be a great-grandparent, or to travel the world, or to live to 100. . . .

Make plans for the future!

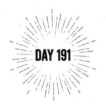

*You will keep in perfect peace those whose minds are steadfast,
because they trust in you. Trust in the Lord forever, for the
Lord, the Lord Himself, is the Rock eternal. . . .
The path of the righteous is level; you, the Upright One,
make the way of the righteous smooth.*

—Isaiah 26:3–4,7 (NIV)

*Heavenly Father, I trust in you. You are my rock. Thank you that
you keep my mind in perfect peace. Thank you that you keep my
path level and that you make my way smooth.*

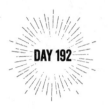

A SURF LESSON

One summer, while on vacation, I paid for a private surf lesson. After multiple spectacular wipeouts, my instructor said something profound.

He said, "Surfing is like life. Don't look back and don't look down. Focus on where you want to go. If you look back, you will lose your balance and fall off. If you look down at your feet, you will lose your balance and fall off. Keep your head up. Pick a point on the shore and look at where you want the board to go. That's how you keep your balance and control the direction of the board." And it worked!

When we look back and focus on the past, we have a tendency to either dwell on our mistakes or wish things were the way they used to be. When we look down at our feet, at our present situation, we tend to get discouraged and depressed and we get stuck.

But when you look ahead and focus on where you want to be, your attitude, outlook, and posture come into alignment. And the things in your life that will help you get there and the things that are not useful are both illuminated.

Don't look back at where you've been. Don't look down at where you are. Focus on where you want to be. Surf's up!

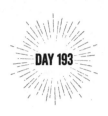

DAY 193

BUT THE PATH OF THE RIGHTEOUS IS LIKE THE LIGHT OF DAWN, THAT SHINES BRIGHTER AND BRIGHTER UNTIL THE FULL DAY.

—PROVERBS 4:18 (NASB)

Heavenly Father, thank you that my path is getting brighter and brighter every day!

JESUS ON WORRY

Therefore, I tell you, do not worry about your life, what you will eat or drink; or about your body, what you will wear. Is not life more than food, and the body more than clothes?

Look at the birds of the air; they do not sow or reap or store away in barns, and yet your heavenly Father feeds them. Are you not much more valuable than they? Can any one of you by worrying add a single hour to your life?

And why do you worry about clothes? See how the flowers of the field grow. They do not labor or spin. Yet I tell you that not even Solomon in all his splendor was dressed like one of these. If that is how God clothes the grass of the field, which is here today and tomorrow is thrown into the fire, will he not much more clothe you—you of little faith?

So do not worry, saying, "What shall we eat?" or "What shall we drink?" or "What shall we wear?" For the pagans run after all these things, and your heavenly Father knows that you need them. But seek first his kingdom and his righteousness, and all these things will be given to you as well.

Therefore, do not worry about tomorrow, for tomorrow will worry about itself. Each day has enough trouble of its own.

—Matthew 6:25–34 (NIV)

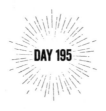

EPIGENETICALLY YOURS

Epigenetics is a branch of science that studies how genes express themselves. It's basically the science of how your choices affect your physical health.

Identical twins carry the same genetics. If one twin gets cancer, the other twin has an increased risk but may never develop cancer. A mutated *BRCA* gene increases a woman's risk of breast cancer, but not every woman with this mutation gets breast cancer. Family history may increase your risk, but your genes don't determine your fate.

You have inherited lots of good genes, and maybe a few bad ones. But you have control over them. You have the power to turn on the cancer-preventing genes and to turn off the cancer-promoting genes in your body!

Your diet, lifestyle, environment, and stress are all factors in whether or not your genes express themselves.

Genetics may load the gun, but your choices pull the trigger. Your choices matter. Make good choices today!

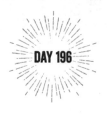

DEATH AND LIFE ARE IN THE POWER OF THE TONGUE, AND THOSE WHO LOVE IT WILL EAT ITS FRUIT.

—PROVERBS 18:21 (NASB)

Your words have the power to create life. So speak life and health to your body. Talk to your organs, bones, and tissues. Encourage them. Give them a pep talk. Tell them you love them. Let each time you remember you have cancer serve as a reminder for you to talk to your body and tell your cancerous cells to be healed and to be well.

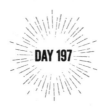

SLOW DOWN

Do you feel like your life has been moving too fast for too long and is now out of your control?

Slow down. Calm down. Slow down your thinking. Slow down your breathing.

Now ask yourself . . .

What things in my life are causing me stress, anxiety, and urgency that I can remove?

Are there obligations, commitments, projects, or demands that I have put on myself that I need to walk away from?

Does the information I consume bring me joy and peace and empower me? Or does it feed my anxiety?

You need peace of mind, peace in your heart, and peace in your body.

Today's Reflection: *Where do you need to apply the brakes?*

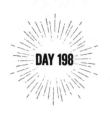

DAY 198

YOU DON'T HAVE TO DIE. YOU CAN GET WELL.

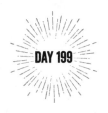

DAY 199

Bless those who persecute you; bless and do not curse. Rejoice with those who rejoice; mourn with those who mourn. Live in harmony with one another. Do not be proud but be willing to associate with people of low position. Do not be conceited.

Do not repay anyone evil for evil. Be careful to do what is right in the eyes of everyone. If it is possible, as far as it depends on you, live at peace with everyone. Do not take revenge, my dear friends, but leave room for God's wrath, for it is written: "It is mine to avenge; I will repay," says the Lord. On the contrary:

"If your enemy is hungry, feed him;

If he is thirsty, give him something to drink.

In doing this, you will heap burning coals on his head."

Do not be overcome by evil but overcome evil with good.

—Romans 12:14–21 (NIV)

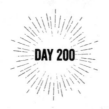

BELIEVE IT'S POSSIBLE

Believe in yourself.

Believe you can get well.

Believe you can survive.

Believe you can beat the odds.

Believe in your body's ability to heal.

Believe that your Heavenly Father has given you everything you need for life and godliness. That He will supply all of your future needs. That He will direct your steps. And that He will deliver you from your affliction.

Jesus said, "All things are possible to him who believes" (Mark 9:23, NASB).

Today's Declaration: *I will survive and thrive. And when I am well, I will help others get well. I believe!*

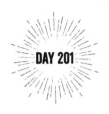

DAY 201

FEED YOUR FAITH
AND STARVE
YOUR FEAR.

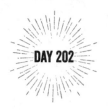

SUCH GREAT FAITH

When Jesus entered Capernaum, a centurion came to Him, imploring Him, and saying, "Lord, my servant is lying paralyzed at home, fearfully tormented."

Jesus said to him, "I will come and heal him."

But the centurion said, "Lord, I am not worthy for You to come under my roof, but just say the word, and my servant will be healed. For I also am a man under authority, with soldiers under me; and I say to this one, 'Go!' and he goes, and to another, 'Come!' and he comes, and to my slave, 'Do this!' and he does it.*"*

Now when Jesus heard this, *He marveled and said to those who were following, "Truly I say to you, I have not found such great faith with anyone in Israel. I say to you that many will come from east and west, and recline* at the table *with Abraham, Isaac and Jacob in the kingdom of heaven; but the sons of the kingdom will be cast out into the outer darkness; in that place there will be weeping and gnashing of teeth."*

And Jesus said to the centurion, "Go; it shall be done for you as you have believed." And the servant was healed that very moment.

—Matthew 8:5–13 (NASB)

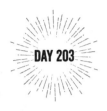

MOTIVATION VERSUS DETERMINATION

The difference between successful people and unsuccessful people is not motivation. Motivation is unpredictable and unreliable. It's easy to take action when you've started something new and exciting. But when the excitement wears off, the motivation often goes with it. And then lack of motivation becomes an excuse for inaction or for not making good choices.

What keeps people going when things get difficult and motivation fades is determination—the force of will inside you that cannot be stopped, no matter what comes against you.

Motivation depends on how you feel in the moment. Determination transcends your feelings and your emotional state. Determination is doing what you know needs to be done, whether you feel like it or not, because you know the end result will be worth the effort and the sacrifice.

Determination is a decision to keep learning, keep doing, keep going, and keep growing until you get what you are after. (This doesn't just apply to health.)

Be determined to make decisions today and every day that move you forward and get you one day closer to where you want to be. #healthyisland

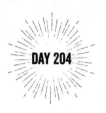

DAY 204

If God is for us, who can be against us? He who did not spare his own Son, but gave him up for us all—how will he not also, along with him, graciously give us all things? Who will bring any charge against those whom God has chosen? It is God who justifies. Who then is the one who condemns? No one. Christ Jesus who died— more than that, who was raised to life—is at the right hand of God and is also interceding for us. Who shall separate us from the love of Christ? Shall trouble or hardship or persecution or famine or nakedness or danger or sword? As it is written:

*"For your sake we face death all day long;
we are considered as sheep to be slaughtered."*

No, in all these things we are more than conquerors through him who loved us. For I am convinced that neither death nor life, neither angels nor demons, neither the present nor the future, nor any powers, neither height nor depth, nor anything else in all creation, will be able to separate us from the love of God that is in Christ Jesus our Lord.

— ROMANS 8:31–39 (NIV)

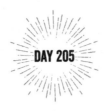

YOU MIGHT HATE THIS, BUT . . .

There is no better way to grow as a person than to do something you hate every day.

—DAVID GOGGINS, *THE TOUGHEST MAN ALIVE*

Maybe it's vegetables. Maybe it's juicing. Maybe it's running. Maybe it's going to the gym. Maybe it's going to bed early. Maybe it's hot saunas. Maybe it's cold showers. Maybe it's meditating. Maybe it's reading. Maybe it's writing. Maybe it's journaling. Maybe it's speaking up. Maybe it's biting your tongue. Maybe it's saying no. Maybe it's admitting when you are wrong. Maybe it's being kind to mean people. Maybe it's forgiveness. . . .

Embrace new things. Embrace change. Embrace challenges. Embrace discomfort. Embrace the things you've avoided. Embrace the things you've been afraid of. Embrace the things you've never liked. Embrace the things you hate to do.

And enjoy growth.

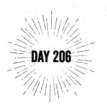

DAY 206

Most of what we say and do is not necessary, and its omission would save both time and trouble. At every step, therefore, a man should ask himself, "Is this one of the things that are superfluous?"

—MARCUS AURELIUS, *MEDITATIONS*

This is a reminder to continue to prune your life. Simplify. Remove the unnecessary to save yourself time and trouble.

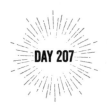

BE QUICK TO FORGIVE

People are going to hurt you. They will be inconsiderate, rude, mean, ugly, cruel, deceptive, abusive, insulting. . . . Some of this will be intentional. Some will be unintentional.

Unless you become a hermit, there's no way to protect yourself from the hurtful words and actions of others. The only thing you have control over is the way you respond.

Imagine if every cut, scrape, or bruise you've had in your life never healed and you had to live with those injuries for the rest of your life. You would be in constant physical pain from head to toe.

If they are not irritated and reinjured, our bodies heal minor injuries. But emotional injuries don't heal on their own. The longer you hold on to an emotional injury, the more damage it does. It's like picking a scab or beating on a bruise so much that it never heals.

Emotional injuries add up over time, leaving you with a battered, bruised, beat-up heart . . . a sick heart.

Bitterness is toxic. The longer you hold on to bitterness, the more damage it does to you. Recognize the injury. Acknowledge the pain. And then forgive right away. Forgiveness heals your heart.

Be quick to forgive.

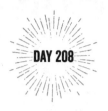

SEE YOURSELF

See yourself healthy.

See yourself whole.

See yourself cancer free.

See yourself happy.

See yourself joyful.

See yourself blessed.

See yourself fulfilled.

See yourself changing the lives of others.

See yourself receiving the desires of your heart.

See yourself dying peacefully at a ripe old age, with your life's mission accomplished.

See yourself standing before your Heavenly Father and hearing the words, "Well done, good and faithful servant!"

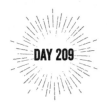

WHAT ARE YOU LOOKING FOR?

If you are looking for things to be upset over and outraged about, you will find them.

If you are looking for things to be thankful for and happy about, you will find them.

The question is: What are you looking for?

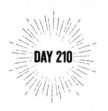

SPEAK TO THE MOUNTAIN

Then Jesus said to the disciples, "Have faith in God. I tell you the truth, you can say to this mountain, 'May you be lifted up and cast into the sea,' and it will happen. But you must really believe it will happen and have no doubt in your heart. I tell you, you can pray for anything, and if you believe that you've received it, it will be yours. But when you are praying, first forgive anyone you are holding a grudge against, so that your Father in heaven will forgive your sins, too."

—MARK 11:22–25 (NLT)

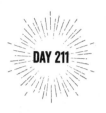

FACE YOUR PROBLEMS HEAD-ON

Don't ignore your problems or pretend they don't exist. You must face your problems head-on because procrastination and problem avoidance will cause more stress and anxiety in your life. The longer you put off your problems, the bigger and more stressful they become.

If you have unresolved problems in your life, they will weigh on your conscious and subconscious mind and lead you to self-medicate with drugs, alcohol, food, and other unhealthy behaviors.

Most of your problems are compartmentalized in your mind—work problems, family problems, health problems—and they feel unrelated. But they're not. Because they are all *your* problems, and your subconscious mind is aware of all of them all the time.

Facing down your problems and working to solve them are vital to stress reduction. As soon as you solve a problem, that stress evaporates. So get busy solving your problems.

Today's Reflection: *What is one problem you've been putting off that you can solve today?*

Action Step: *Make a to-do list of every problem that you need to solve.*

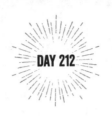

DAY 212

PEACE DOES NOT MEAN TO BE IN A PLACE WHERE THERE IS NO NOISE, TROUBLE, OR HARD WORK. IT MEANS TO BE IN THE MIDST OF THOSE THINGS AND STILL BE CALM IN YOUR HEART.

—UNKNOWN

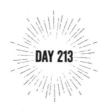

WALKING CAN SAVE YOUR LIFE!

All exercise is great, but the most underestimated form of exercise is walking.

A study of nearly 140,000 Americans found that just 150 minutes a week of brisk walking was linked to a 20 percent reduction in death from all causes!

A U.K. study of over 50,000 people came to the same conclusion, and also found that walking was associated with a 24 percent reduced risk of dying from cardiovascular disease, like a heart attack or stroke.[29]

Brisk walking is walking at a deliberately quick pace that might get you a bit out of breath after a few minutes. Think of it as walking with purpose. One hundred fifty minutes of brisk walking a week breaks down to 20 to 30 minutes per day, which is about a mile or two.

Make it fun! Walk the dog, walk with friends or family, or walk by yourself to get some alone time. Call someone you haven't talked to in a while. Or listen to music or a podcast or an audio book. Or listen to Johnny Cash reading the New Testament. Trust me; it's awesome.

An easy way to make walking a part of your daily routine is to walk for 10 to 15 minutes after lunch and dinner. Just walk every day. Movement is life!

29 Stmatakas et al., "Self-Rated Walking Pace and All-Cause, Cardiovascular Disease and Cancer Mortality: Individual Participant Pooled Analysis of 50 225 Walkers from 11 Population British Cohorts," *British Journal of Sports Medicine* 52, no. 12 (June 2018): 761–768.

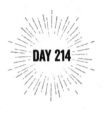

YOU HAVE DIVINE DIRECTION

*The Lord directs the steps of the godly. He delights in every
detail of their lives. Though they stumble, they will
never fall, for the Lord holds them by the hand.*

—PSALM 37:23–24 (NLT)

*Father, thank You that You direct my steps, thank You for caring
about every detail of my life, thank You for holding me by the hand
on this journey, and thank You that You will never let me fall!*

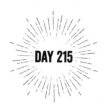

Healing is like a roller-coaster ride. You can be sure you will have up days, down days, and upside-down days. Be prepared and anticipate the twists and turns. How you respond is key!

Build your healing team, write out your perfect day, and make a healing plan. Have plans in place for bad days and scan days. This is your journey; all of your teams and plans must be customized for you! Create the best plan for you.

Your healing team should consist of your practitioners, coaches, friends, family, encouragers, and prayer warriors. Your team should only include people who believe in your approach and, most importantly, believe in you!

You will have those days when you just don't feel good physically and/or emotionally. Your bad-day plan should include calls to your encouragers, coach check-ins, breathing exercises, Emotional Freedom Techniques (EFT), sunshine, worship, extra time with God, and rest . . . to name a few. All of these things help turn a bad day around.

Heal your heart, forgive, let things go, laugh, and *love* big. My prayer is for your total healing in Jesus's name.

Never lose hope, my hero!

—*Tara Mann, founder of Cancer Crackdown*[30]

---

30 Cancer Crackdown is a nonprofit organization that helps cancer patients find natural and alternative healing therapies. Connect with Tara Mann at www.cancercrackdown.org.

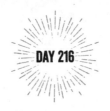

YOU ARE BECOMING A GENIUS

When you decide to do something that most people would never dream of doing, people are going to think you are crazy.

Don't worry about the people who don't understand you.

Eventually most of them will because . . .

Time changes things.

According to NBA legend Mike Newlin, "Genius is perseverance in disguise."

And to paraphrase Thomas Carlyle, "Genius is the infinite capacity for dealing with trouble."

Genius is the ability to persevere through your troubles.

And while you persevere, look forward to the future: to success, triumph, and glory.

People who called you crazy in the beginning will eventually call you a genius.

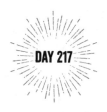

TIME IS YOUR MOST VALUABLE ASSET

When you work, you trade your time for money.

If you spend your money, you can always trade more time for more money.

But time spent can never be bought back.

Life is precious, and time is short.

Invest your time in experiences, things, and people that matter.

Spend your time wisely. Don't waste it.

Time is your most valuable asset.

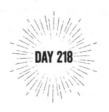

NO ONE TALKS TO YOU MORE THAN YOU

Instead of depending on encouragement from others, which may be in short supply, now is the time to be your own head coach and start encouraging yourself.

You can apply this to every area of your life. *I am smart. I am strong. I am courageous. I am loved. I am worthy of love. I am blessed. I am attractive. I am successful. I am valuable. I belong here. I can do this. I am healed. I am healthy. I am well.*

Talk to your body. Talk to your organs. Talk to your cancer cells. Tell them you love them. Tell them to be healed. And tell them to be well.

Taking care of your physical body with healthy food and exercise is one way to love yourself. But the most important way to love yourself is also choosing to think about yourself and speak to yourself in a loving, kind, and encouraging way. This requires daily practice and may feel strange at first.

If you've been in the habit of beating yourself up and even hating yourself, stop doing that. Interrupt those critical self-defeating thoughts with loving encouragement and the affirmations above.

Today's Challenge: *Encourage yourself and talk to your body.*

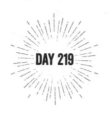

WHEN WE ARE NO LONGER ABLE TO CHANGE A SITUATION . . . WE ARE CHALLENGED TO CHANGE OURSELVES.

—VIKTOR FRANKL

The path to healing begins by changing yourself.
Changing yourself changes your situation.
Accept the challenge to change yourself!

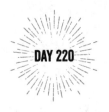

VICTIM OR VICTOR?

*But thanks be to God! He gives us the victory through
our Lord Jesus Christ.*

—1 Corinthians 15:57 (NIV)

No one wants to be a victim. And anyone can be victimized
in a moment. But many of us choose to operate in a perpetual state of victimhood. This is a state of powerlessness,
helplessness, and hopelessness.

Being a victor is a choice.

The attitude of a victor is one of determination to triumph over adversity.

The victim says, "Things happen to me."

The victor says, "Things happen for me."

Challenges in life happen to make you smarter, stronger, wiser, more patient, more flexible, more resilient, more
kind, more compassionate, more loving, more like Jesus, the
ultimate Victor.

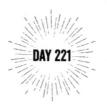

DAY 221

*Progress . . . is not achieved by accident or luck,
but by working on yourself—daily.*

—EPICTETUS, *ART OF LIVING*

You are a work in progress. Each day gives you the opportunity to improve, grow, and heal. Even though you may not see or feel changes every day, you are changing for the better. Progress is happening. Believe it!

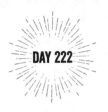

DO YOU WANNA BUILD A SNOWMAN?

My hometown (Memphis, Tennessee) only gets a few days of snow each year. And if you want to make a snowman, you'd better do it on day 1—the first day of snow—because most of the snow will be melted in 36 hours.

In order to build a snowman, first you make a tiny snowball with your hands. Then you start rolling it around on the ground. And as you roll, it gradually picks up more snow and gets bigger. This takes more work than you remember. You pick up a lot of sticks and leaves and dirt along the way, and it doesn't look good. Your little helpers get tired and go inside, but you can't just leave a big dirty snowball in the front yard. Then all the neighbors will see that you're a snowman-building failure. So you keep going.

The healing journey is kind of like building a snowman. It takes patience and persistence, and it is hard work. You may feel like you're out in the cold with no help. You may feel like no one cares. But you can see the end result. And that's why you keep going. Once the hard work is done and you've built your snowman, you can pick all the leaves and sticks and dirt out, shape it, smooth it out, and put the finishing touches on your masterpiece.

Don't stop. Don't quit. Keep rolling that snowball.

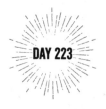

WORRY AND DOUBT ARE THE OPPOSITE OF FAITH

Exercising your faith means trusting God to lead you, protect you, provide for you, and heal you. You can't be in faith and worrying at the same time. Fully trusting Him means letting go of fear—choosing to believe and not to doubt.

As part of my daily routine, every time I felt worried and afraid, this is what I prayed:

> *Lord, I am not going to be afraid. I am giving you my fear. Jesus, I am laying it at your feet. I trust you with my life, my health, my family, my finances, my future. I trust you. Thank you for leading me in the path of healing, for supplying all of my needs, and for working everything out for my good. Amen.*

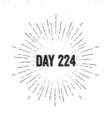

DAY 224

IF YOU CARE ABOUT SOMEONE ELSE'S HEALTH MORE THAN THEY DO, YOU PROBABLY CAN'T HELP THEM.

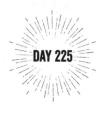

THE LOVE BANK

My wife, Micah, and I have been married for 19 years, and something we learned early on that has helped us stay together is a concept called the Love Bank.

When someone is kind to you, compliments you, buys you gifts, shows you affection, or serves you in some way, they make a deposit into your Love Bank. And your love for them grows. And when you do those kinds of things for another person, you make a deposit into their Love Bank and their love for *you* grows.

But if you're critical of them, if you're mean, if you ignore them, if you neglect them, you make withdrawals from their Love Bank. And you know what happens if you make too many withdrawals from the bank? Eventually your account goes to zero. Then it goes negative.

Most relationships fail because one or both parties selfishly make more withdrawals than deposits, and eventually their accounts become overdrawn and the love is gone.

If someone in your life is constantly complaining about certain things you do, you can be sure that those things are making withdrawals from their Love Bank.

Action Step #1: Stop doing the things that drain your loved one's Love Bank.

Action Step #2: Transform your relationships by making Love Bank deposits every day, and watch their love for you grow![31]

---

31 Recommended reading: *His Needs, Her Needs: Building an Affair-Proof Marriage* by Willard F. Harley, Jr.

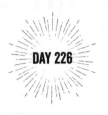

THE FIVE LOVE LANGUAGES

According to best-selling author Gary Chapman, there are five ways we give and receive love, which he calls *The Five Love Languages:* words of affirmation, acts of service, receiving gifts, quality time, and physical touch.

We each have one or two love languages that make us feel most loved, and we often give love in the way we want to receive it. But this may not be how someone else feels most loved. . . . Think of the love languages as different denominations of currency. For some, a thoughtful gift makes a $5 deposit in their Love Bank, but an act of service makes a $20 deposit.

Telling my wife that I love her, helping with housework, buying her flowers, going for walks with her, and hugging her all make deposits into her Love Bank. But her main love languages are quality time and acts of service. And they make the biggest deposits. If I constantly told my wife I loved her and bought her gifts, but was always gone and never helped with the house or the kids, I would not be meeting her most important needs. And by neglecting those needs, I would end up making larger withdrawals than deposits, and our relationship would suffer.

Here's your action plan. Figure out the love languages of your loved ones so you can love them in the way they feel most loved. And make sure you communicate your love languages to them so that they can love you back in the best way. And maximize those Love Bank deposits![32]

---

32 Recommended reading: *The Five Love Languages* by Gary Chapman

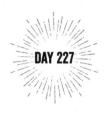

HE WHO IS SLOW TO ANGER IS BETTER THAN THE MIGHTY, AND HE WHO RULES HIS SPIRIT, [IS BETTER] THAN HE WHO CAPTURES A CITY.

—PROVERBS 16:32 (NASB)

Anger suppresses your immune system. And we make bad choices when we are angry.

Today's Challenge: *Rule your spirit. If someone or something provokes you to anger, catch yourself in that split second before you react and choose a peaceful, patient, loving response. Or choose not to respond.*

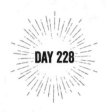

THREE SECRETS OF LONG LIFE

Okinawa has the highest percentage of centenarians—people who live to at least 100—in the world. And here are three secrets of their longevity.

Secret #1 is a concept known as *hara hachi bu*. This is a cultural practice that means you stop eating when you are 80 percent full. This a great strategy to lose weight and stay trim. But if you need to gain weight, eat more.

Secret #2 is having a *moai*. Your moai is your tribe, the people you love, share common interests with, and spend time with. Isolation promotes depression and disease. We need each other. We need real-world connection and community. Spend as much time as possible with your moai.

Secret #3 is *ikigai*, which means having a sense of purpose in life: a reason for living, the thing that gets you out of bed in the morning. In many countries, people retire in their 60s and then their health starts to decline. But in Japan the concept of retirement doesn't exist! And in Okinawa a person's ikigai often grows as they get older. Ikigai is especially important for cancer patients. Identify your reasons to live. Focus on them. And let that motivate you in your healing journey.

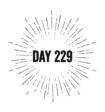

DAY 229

Here's a wonderful affirmation from Louise Hay:

ALL IS WELL. EVERYTHING IS WORKING OUT FOR MY HIGHEST GOOD. OUT OF THIS SITUATION ONLY GOOD WILL COME. I AM SAFE.

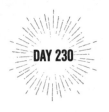

LET IT GO

It's time to clean house. Not just your figurative house—your body—but also your literal house. Owning too much stuff is a burden and can be a significant source of smoldering stress. Marketers have convinced us that our possessions define us, but they don't. They enslave us. The more you have, the more you have to take care of. And then what you own ends up owning you!

Get rid of the clutter. Reduce your load. And free yourself from the burden of stuff. Clean out your cabinets. Clean out your closets. Clean out your attic. Clean out the garage. Clean out the storage unit. Real talk: If you haven't worn it or used it in years, you ain't gonna! Stop holding on to stuff from the past. As they say, "You can't take it with you." So let it go.

Sell your stuff online if you need some extra cash or donate it to charity (this is much quicker and easier).

You may have a lot to do, but don't get overwhelmed. Start with a small area that won't take long, like a cluttered kitchen cabinet. When that's done, you're going to feel really good. Then move on to the other cabinets, then one closet at a time, then your garage, then your attic. Make a list and work through it. You can do this!

Today's Challenge: *Clean out a cabinet and make a to-do list to tackle the rest.*

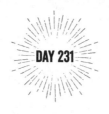

DAY 231

STAY AWAY FROM NEGATIVE PEOPLE. THEY HAVE A PROBLEM FOR EVERY SOLUTION.

—ANONYMOUS

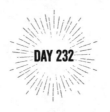

HOW TO TELL IF YOU HAD A GREAT DAY

Every day you aren't filing for divorce or bankruptcy is a great day.

Every day you aren't being evicted from your home is a great day.

Every day you aren't standing on a street corner with a sign asking for money is a great day.

Every day you aren't wondering where your next meal will come from is a great day.

Every day you aren't wondering where you will sleep is a great day.

Every day you aren't sitting in jail for a crime you didn't commit is a great day.

Every day you aren't considering prostitution to make ends meet is a great day.

Every day you aren't burying someone you love is a great day.

Every day you aren't lying in a hospital bed dying is a great day.

So how's today looking?

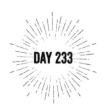

IF YOU'RE AFRAID, DO IT AFRAID.

—JOYCE MEYER, *DO IT AFRAID!*

It's easy to think that you shouldn't do something because you feel scared. But courage can only manifest in the midst of fear. Don't let fear and all the "what-ifs" paralyze you and keep you from doing what you want to do and what you need to do. You are strong. You are not alone. Be brave. Push through your fear. Triumph and blessings are on the other side.

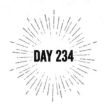

DAY 234

*To most people nothing is more troublesome than
the effort of thinking.*

—JAMES BRYCE

It's much easier to have someone else do your thinking for you and to tell you what to do and what not to do. That's what we are conditioned for and it's what most of us prefer. But living that way makes you powerless. It's like handing someone else the keys to your car. And right now, more than ever, you need to be in the driver's seat of your life and healing journey. You need to put your problem-solving brain to work. You may be facing major decisions with life-and-death consequences. Think them through carefully. If you don't understand what is being recommended to you, if it doesn't make sense, don't blindly say yes. You need more time to read, research, learn, and think.

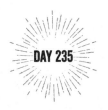

JUST LIKE A VIRUS, FEAR MUST ALSO RUN ITS COURSE

*God has not given us a spirit of fear, but of power
and of love and of a sound mind.*

—2 TIMOTHY 1:7 (NKJV)

Fear is highly contagious. If you are surrounded by fearful people and you are paying attention to people who are spreading fear on TV or online, they will infect you with fear.

And once infected with fear, you will become irrational. And you will make impulsive, fear-based decisions, which are almost always the wrong ones.

Some people, even doctors, will try to use fear as a weapon against you, to control you and manipulate you. Don't let them.

A sound mind is a rational mind. A rational person does not rush into things, or panic, or let fear or a sense of urgency cloud their judgment. A rational mind acknowledges fear, addresses it head-on, and makes wise, thoughtful, well-reasoned decisions. A rational person trusts God to lead them.

The antidote to fear is faith.

Your Heavenly Father will protect you and provide for you.

So give your worries and fears to God today, and trust Him with your life and your future.

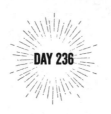

DAY 236

BITTERNESS IS POISON. FORGIVENESS IS THE ANTIDOTE.

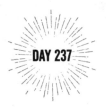

DAY 237

Take a deep breath. Get present in the moment and ask yourself what is important this very second.

—GREG MCKEOWN, AUTHOR OF *ESSENTIALISM*

It's easy to get busy and distracted and to fill up an entire day with trivial and meaningless activities that don't get you any closer to your goals. Every day you have a to-do list and you must prioritize the items on that list. The things you want to do most are not necessarily the things you need to do. And oftentimes we make excuses and convince ourselves that the trivial tasks are more essential than they really are. Stop doing that. When faced with the choice on what to do next, ask yourself: *What is the most important thing I should be doing right now?* And do that thing.

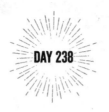

DAY 238

In his letter to the church in Philippi, the Apostle Paul shares the secret of being content. Keep in mind that Paul wrote this while imprisoned in Rome and facing execution for spreading the message that Jesus Christ was the Messiah and Savior of the world.

> *I have learned to be content whatever the circumstances. I know what it is to be in need, and I know what it is to have plenty. I have learned the secret of being content in any and every situation, whether well fed or hungry, whether living in plenty or in want. I can do all this through him [Christ] who gives me strength.*
> —Philippians 4:11–13 (NIV)

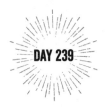

DAY 239

He is a wise man who does not grieve for the things which he has not, but rejoices for those which he has.

—Anonymous, often attributed to Epictetus

Focusing on what you don't have fills you with envy and misery. Focusing on what you do have fills you with gratitude. I love that this quote says rejoice for what you have. Count your blessings and rejoice; show great joy and delight in what you have!

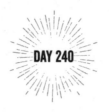

NOT DOING THIS IS WORSE THAN SMOKING

A 2018 study conducted at the Cleveland Clinic, which followed 122,000 people for 23 years, found that not exercising is worse for your health than smoking!

The researchers found that those who engaged in high levels of exercise lived longer, healthier lives.

According to study coauthor Dr. Wael Jaber, "Being unfit on a treadmill or an exercise stress test has a worse prognosis as far as death than being hypertensive (high blood pressure), being diabetic, or being a current smoker. We've never seen something as pronounced and as objective as this."[33]

The people who were in the worst physical shape at the beginning of the study had the highest risk of death over the next 20 years. And the people who were in the best physical shape had the lowest risk of death.[34] So let's get in shape!

Running, rowing, rebounding, swimming, biking, jazzercise, Zumba, rock climbing . . . It doesn't matter what type of exercise you do. It's all good! Do something that you enjoy for 30 to 60 minutes per day, 6 days a week.

This is a loving reminder from me to you to exercise today.

33 Gina Martinez, "Not Exercising May Be Worse for Your Health Than Smoking, Study Says," *Time*, October 2, 2018, https://time.com/5430203/new-study-not-exercising-worse
-than-smoking/.
34 Mandsager et al., "Association of Cardiorespiratory Fitness with Long-Term Mortality Among Adults Undergoing Exercise Treadmill Testing," *JAMA Network* 1, no. 2 (Oct 19, 2018): e183605.

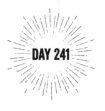

DAY 241

Growth and comfort do not coexist.
—GINNI ROMETTY

The desire to stay in your comfort zone is rooted in fear. But comfort leads to stagnation, regression, entropy, weakness, and decay. If you want to grow as a person, to grow in health, to grow in wisdom and knowledge, and to grow in your relationships, embrace new uncomfortable things. New things make you uncomfortable because you don't understand them. You don't know what you are doing, maybe because you're afraid of failure and looking foolish. But that's okay! Push yourself out of your comfort zone, because discomfort stimulates growth. Now is your time for growth!

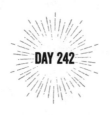

HUMBLE YOURSELVES UNDER THE MIGHTY HAND OF GOD, THAT HE MAY EXALT YOU AT THE PROPER TIME, CASTING ALL YOUR ANXIETY ON HIM, BECAUSE HE CARES FOR YOU.

—1 PETER 5:6–7 (NASB)

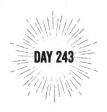

SOMETIMES THE BEST THING TO DO IS NOTHING

Fasting is one of the most powerful therapies because it increases cellular detoxification and regenerates your immune system.

During a fast, you will experience physical withdrawal and cravings for addictive foods. And as your body breaks down fat for energy, toxins stored in fat are released, which may make you feel bad. Some common reactions are low energy, headaches, nausea, or aches and pains. You could break out in a rash, throw up, have diarrhea, or even run a fever. These symptoms are not unusual and are known as a *healing crisis*. Even though it feels unpleasant, good things are happening.

I recommend you start a fast on a Friday. That way, the hardest days (days two and three) fall on the weekend. Clear your schedule and plan to rest on the days you may feel lousiest. Stay in bed if you need to. When you get over the detoxification hump, usually on day four, you may be surprised by how good you feel, considering the fact that you haven't eaten in days.

There is an exponential benefit to fasting for three days versus one or two days. And those benefits continue to increase over days four and five. Consider a three- to five-day fast every month or two as part of your healing strategy.

Fasting is generally safe for most people, but you should consult your doctor before attempting a fast.

DAY 244

IF YOU LIVE AND EAT THE WAY EVERYONE ELSE DOES, YOU CAN EXPECT TO GET THE SAME CHRONIC DISEASES EVERYONE GETS.

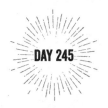

GO OUTSIDE

Leave everything inside for a moment. Your worries, your fears, your problems, your phone . . . not your clothes.

Now it's just you, outside in the world. Feel the air. Is it warm or cool? Is there wind? Is it still? Smell the air. What do you smell?

Stand up straight. Breathe deeply. Stretch.

Look at your surroundings. Survey the landscape. What do you see? Look at the trees, flowers, and plants. Listen for birds and insects. Look for them in the trees and bushes. Look at the sky. Where is the sun? Are there clouds?

Take your shoes off and feel the dirt, the grass, the sand, or the rocks with your toes.

This world was created for you, and you for it.

Marvel at the miraculous and infinite complexity and beauty of nature.

You are a tiny little thing on a huge planet, and yet your Heavenly Father cares about every aspect of your life.

You are alive. And you are infinitely loved.

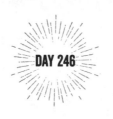

DO NOT BE WISE IN YOUR OWN EYES; FEAR THE LORD AND TURN AWAY FROM EVIL. IT WILL BE HEALING TO YOUR BODY AND REFRESHMENT TO YOUR BONES.

—PROVERBS 3:7–8 (NASB)

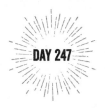

NOW IS THE TIME

Now is the time to be adventurous.

Now is the time to pioneer uncharted territory.

Now is the time to "Boldly go where no man has gone before."

Okay, maybe not that far . . .

Now is the time to boldly go where *you* have never gone before.

Now is the time to let go of the past.

Now is the time to embrace the present.

Now is the time to plan for the future.

Now is the time to take the wheel of your life and hit the road.

Now is the time to do things you've always wanted to do, the things you've been putting off.

Now is the time to say, "Why not?"

Now is your time to live!

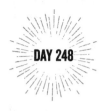

ALL THINGS FOR YOUR GOOD

Consider that things which happen in life are happening for you, not to you. And by for you, I mean for your good.

That doesn't mean bad things are okay. Of course they aren't.

But there is a promise in Scripture that God will use the bad things for good.

In his letter to the Roman church, the Apostle Paul wrote, "And we know that God causes all things to work together for good to those who love God, to those who are called according to His purpose" (Romans 8:28, NASB).

Before Paul wrote that, he had been imprisoned numerous times and whipped with 39 lashes (the legal limit) five times. He had been beaten with rods three times. He had been stoned, dragged out of the city, and left for dead. He had been shipwrecked three times and spent a day and night adrift at sea, presumably floating on a piece of a wrecked ship! In his travels to spread the Gospel, Paul had been in constant danger from other people as well as in the wild, and had been through many sleepless nights, hungry and thirsty and suffering in the cold.

When Paul said that God works all things for the good of those who love Him, he meant *all* things! Believe it!

Father, thank you for working all things for my good.

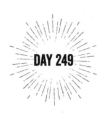
DAY 249

PLANS FAIL WHERE THERE IS NO COUNSEL, BUT WITH MANY ADVISERS THEY SUCCEED.

—PROVERBS 15:22 (HCSB)

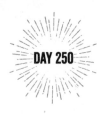

LEARN FROM SUCCESSFUL PEOPLE

You don't know it all. And you don't need to.

But you need to learn more. Because what you learn could change your life, or even save your life. So it's time to "go back to school."

Do you want to be successful in your endeavors? Don't wait to be told what to do. Find successful people, learn from them, and do what they do.

Don't let envy or jealousy or pride get in the way. Successful people are pioneers. Don't resent them. Be thankful for them, because their success can help you create your own.

The help you need is closer than you think. There are people who have already done what you are trying to do. Find them. Study them. And imitate them. Your path will be different from theirs, but the wisdom and knowledge you can glean from them will be invaluable to you.

If you are trying to heal cancer, go to chrisbeatcancer .com and watch the Survivor Interviews. They will encourage you and inspire you and give you fresh ideas and resources you didn't know existed. Type your cancer type into the search bar and see who and what comes up.

Today's Challenge: *Make a decision to find and learn from successful people.*

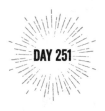

DAY 251

And if the Spirit of him who raised Jesus from the dead is living in you, he who raised Christ from the dead will also give life to your mortal bodies through his Spirit who lives in you.

—Romans 8:11 (NASB)

Memorize this Scripture. Meditate on it and confess it over your life and your situation:

The Holy Spirit of God who raised Jesus from the dead dwells in me and gives life to my body today!

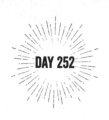

DAY 252

**YOUR PAIN BECOMES
YOUR PURPOSE.**

**YOUR MESS BECOMES
YOUR MESSAGE.**

**YOUR TEST BECOMES
YOUR TESTIMONY.**

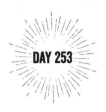

DAY 253

Courage is resistance to fear, mastery of fear—not absence of fear.

—MARK TWAIN

There are moments throughout the day when you are so thoroughly preoccupied by something—work, exercise, conversation, music, a show, or a movie—that you are blissfully unaware that you have cancer. And it's wonderful. But inevitably, you remember. And a wave of fear washes over you.

Fear is a persistent foe. And at the beginning of the cancer journey, it's intense and it's close, persistently trying to hijack your thoughts and emotions. Take heart, dear one, your fear will diminish over time, but until then, you must resist it. At every opportunity, give your worries and fears to your Heavenly Father. Trust Him with your life, your health, your family, and your future. Be courageous. Resist and master your fear.

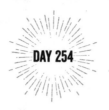

DAY 254

GONNA MAKE YOU SWEAT!

You know that sweating helps cool you off when you're hot. But did you know that sweating is your body's best way to detoxify many heavy metals like mercury, aluminum, cadmium, copper, and lead?

A study comparing the excretion of heavy metals in sweat versus urine found that sweating detoxified 52 times more copper, 25 times more manganese, 13 times more nickel and uranium, 11 times more cadmium and lead, 5 times more aluminum, and 20 percent more mercury than urine.[35] That's legit!

But if you aren't sweating regularly, you may not be sufficiently detoxifying these heavy metals from your body.

The study also found that, with the exception of lead, more heavy metals were excreted from sauna sweating than from sweaty exercise.

Some people hate to exercise and hate to sweat, and avoid both at all costs. If that's you, learn to love them both. They are so good for you!

Get some sweaty exercise five to six days a week. And if you can afford to buy a sauna or have access to a sauna (not a steam room) at your local gym, work in 10 to 20 minutes of sauna sweating to accelerate heavy metal detoxification.

35 Stephen Genuis, Ilia Rodushkin, and Sanjay Beesoon, "Blood, Urine, and Sweat (BUS) Study: Monitoring and Elimination of Bioaccumulated Toxic Elements," *Archives of Environmental Contamination and Toxicology* 61 (November 6, 2011): 344–357. https://www.academia.edu/30142616/Blood_Urine_and_Sweat_BUS_Study_Monitoring_and_Elimination_of_Bioaccumulated_Toxic_Elements.

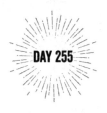

DAY 255

*Surely He has borne our griefs
And carried our sorrows;
Yet we esteemed Him stricken,
Smitten by God, and afflicted.
But He was wounded for our transgressions,
He was bruised for our iniquities;
The chastisement for our peace was upon Him,
And by His stripes we are healed*

—Isaiah 53:4–5 (NKJV)

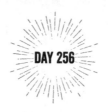

SMALL CHANGE ADDS UP

Massive action produces massive results.

But massive action doesn't just mean making big changes.

Taking massive action means you will be making big changes, for sure. But it also means you will be making a lot of small changes too.

Big changes often have a measurable impact right away, which is great. But over time all of the small changes you make to your life could have as much as, or even more of, an impact than the handful of big changes you make. In statistics, this phenomenon is called the "long tail."

In other words, half of your results may come from 20 percent of your actions (the big changes) and the other half may come from the other 80 percent of your actions (all the small changes).

The little things matter. So don't neglect the small things.

Pull the big levers and the small levers.

All those small changes add up to massive results!

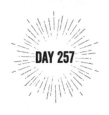

THE FEAR OF THE LORD PROLONGS LIFE, BUT THE YEARS OF THE WICKED ARE CUT SHORT.

—PROVERBS 10:27 (HCSB)

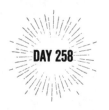

GROW TIME

*God Almighty first planted a garden; and, indeed,
it is the purest of human pleasures.*

—Francis Bacon, *Essays, Civil and Moral*

Gardening is hardwired into our nature as humans. We are all gardeners at heart.

If you've never done it, or aren't currently doing it, I want to encourage you to grow some food.

Very few things connect you to nature more than creating a garden: sowing seeds, tending to them daily, and watching them grow. The time you spend outside in the fresh air and sunshine tending to your plants is immensely therapeutic. And then, enjoying your super nutritious, freshly grown produce at harvest time is especially gratifying.

You could start with a small container garden on your porch or patio, or you could invest in an aeroponic Tower Garden®, or you could build some raised beds in your yard. We've done all of the above!

Grow tomatoes, potatoes, carrots, lettuce, garlic, onions, kale, spinach, cucumbers, squash, peppers, and herbs (like cilantro, rosemary, basil, and dill). Plant some fruit trees or berry bushes. You are a gardener. Grow things!

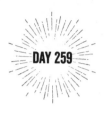

DAY 259

THE FEARS OF THE WICKED WILL BE FULFILLED; THE HOPES OF THE GODLY WILL BE GRANTED. WHEN THE STORMS OF LIFE COME, THE WICKED ARE WHIRLED AWAY, BUT THE GODLY HAVE A LASTING FOUNDATION.

—PROVERBS 10:24–25 (NLV)

Father, thank you that my hopes will be granted and that I have a lasting foundation to weather every storm of life!

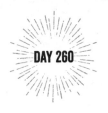

BREATHE DEEPLY

Deep, controlled breathing activates the relaxation response in your body. It calms down your nervous system, lowers stress, releases tension, quiets your scattered mind, and puts you back in control.

Here is a simple deep breathing exercise you can incorporate into your daily healing routine to relieve stress.

Sit comfortably. Close your eyes. Take a deep breath through your nose. Pause for a moment. Then exhale through your nose as slowly as possible, as if you were pinching the opening of a balloon. As you exhale, let yourself melt, releasing any tension you are holding in your body. Pause at the bottom. And repeat.

Be still. Pay attention to the miraculous body that God gave you, and listen to your breath. Feel the air come in through your nose. Listen to the sound it makes. Feel your lungs expand. Visualize the oxygen going through your lungs to your heart. As you exhale, feel your lungs gently deflate. And listen to the sound of your breath leaving your body. Feel your heart beat. When you notice your mind wandering—it eventually will—just bring your attention back to your breath.

Today's Challenge: *Twenty deep, controlled breaths. Count on the exhale.*

This will take 5 to 6 minutes. Then see how you feel. If you feel good, keep going! Meditative deep breathing for 10 to 20 minutes per day is ideal to maximize the benefits.

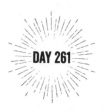

DAY 261

What we fear doing most is usually what we most need to do.

—Tim Ferriss, *The 4-Hour Workweek*

The thing you want to do the least—the thing you're really, really avoiding—is usually the thing you need to do the most.

Problem avoidance leads to stress.

Stress leads to self-medication.

Self-medication is typically achieved through unhealthy and destructive behavior: smoking, drinking, drug use, gambling, overeating, overworking, sex addiction, shopping addiction, binge-watching, gaming, escapism . . .

And those unhealthy behaviors all contribute to disease.

Doing the things that you fear is the most powerful way to extinguish those fears and root out the underlying causes of your stress and anxiety.

Today's Reflection: *What is that thing that you fear, that you are avoiding, that you need to address head-on today?*

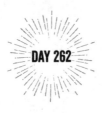

DAY 262

Jesus said, "But I say love your enemies! Pray for those who persecute you! In that way, you will be acting as true children of your Father in heaven."

—MATTHEW 5:44–45 (NLT)

If you stand up for anything, you will have opposition. People will decide to be your enemy. And they will attack you and treat you unfairly. This cannot be avoided. You cannot control what others do, but you can control what you do in response.

You can choose to love your enemies.

Loving your enemies is hard. No one wants to do this. You want to defend yourself. You want to fight back.

Just because someone decides to be your enemy, that doesn't mean you have to be theirs.

Choosing to love your enemies by praying for them and blessing them is letting go of the conflict and giving it to God. This is exactly what Jesus did when his enemies nailed Him to a cross. He said, "Father forgive them for they know not what they do."

So today is a reminder to pray for your enemies. Forgive them. Pray that God reveals Himself to them, ask Him to change their hearts, and ask Him to bless them. And ask Him to show you how you can show love and kindness to them.

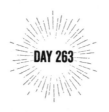

DAY 263

DON'T QUIT

There's a point in every prolonged endeavor when excitement and enthusiasm fade. Your energy and confidence are depleted. Mental and physical exhaustion increase. You second-guess your decisions. You question your beliefs. Your faith is tested. And discouragement and depression loom.

What was easy in the beginning now feels hard. You're not sure if the sacrifice was worth it. The end seems far away. You don't know if you will make it. You feel completely alone. You've hit the wall.

And you want to call it quits.

This is the dark night of the soul, where the pressure to give up is the most intense. It's the ultimate test of your faith, your determination, your fortitude, and your resolve. And this is where many people quit.

I am at that point now in writing this book. And you may be at this point in your journey. So I will tell you what I tell myself.

This is bigger than you. You must press on. You've come too far to stop. The night is always darkest just before the dawn. The light is coming. Picture yourself crossing the finish line, victorious. Feel that feeling of triumph and elation. The effort and sacrifice will be worth it.

Don't quit!

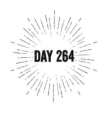

DAY 264

But the fruit of the Spirit is love, joy, peace, patience, kindness, goodness, faithfulness, gentleness, self-control.

—Galatians 5:22–23 (NASB)

The more you become like Jesus, the more good fruit you produce in your life. . . .

You become more loving—caring, not indifferent to others.

You become more joyful—happy, not moody or grumpy.

You become more peaceful—at ease, not filled with anxiety or worry.

You become more patient—calm, not rushed or short-tempered.

You become more kind—not rude, cruel, or critical.

You become "more good"—honest, moral, and ethical.

You become more faithful—hopeful, optimistic, reliable, and not cynical.

You become gentler—not harsh, abrasive, and aggressive.

You exercise more self-control—not impulsive, irresponsible, and unorganized.

Today's Reflection: *Which of these fruits need more cultivation in your life? And how can you act differently today?*

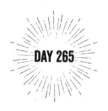
WHAT YOU FOCUS ON EXPANDS

If you focus on your problems—on the things you lack, the things you want but don't have, the people who've hurt you, and the mistakes in your past—your unhappiness will expand.

But if you focus on joy, happiness, love, and gratitude, *they* will expand in your life. Focus on the present and on the things in your life that make your life worth living and on the things you can do today to improve your health and make your life better.

When I was diagnosed with cancer, I had every reason to be negative, bitter, angry, and jealous of healthy people. And I was, at first.

But cancer taught me how to fully trust God to work all things for my good, how to exercise gratitude, how to be thankful, how to be content, how to focus on all the good things in my life instead of the bad, and how to find joy in my most difficult season of life.

The worst thing that has ever happened to me has made my life more fulfilling than I could ever have imagined.

Cancer changed me for the better and it can do the same for you.

What you focus on expands.

NO ONE, NOT EVEN YOUR DOCTOR, HAS THE POWER OR AUTHORITY TO PREDICT THE END OF YOUR LIFE, UNLESS YOU GIVE IT TO THEM.

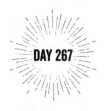

WRITE YOUR STORY

If you think I'm going to tell you to write down everything that's happening to you because it could turn into an article or a book or a course or a movie one day . . . you're right. I am.

But I'm also telling you to do something that's much bigger than journaling or keeping a diary.

You see, whether you write it down or not, every day of your life is a page in your story. Your thoughts, decisions, and actions each day write your life story.

Maybe your life story up to this point stinks. Maybe it's page after page of anger, resentment, unhappiness, jealousy, conflict, abuse, self-medication, and self-sabotage. Or maybe it's boring and unfulfilling and nothing ever happens.

If you don't like the way your life story is going, it's time to write a new story.

You can write a story of love, courage, hope, adventure, success, risk and reward, triumph, and healing. Your story could take you around the country or around the world.

You can become the hero of your story, instead of the victim.

Write your new story.

And write it down.

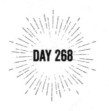

FEAR INTO ACTION

Fear can motivate you in one of two directions: courage or cowardice.

Every soldier on the battlefield is afraid.

No one feels courageous, because courage isn't a feeling.

Fear is the feeling.

Cowardice is the decision to abandon your post, to run away, to hide, to break your commitment.

Courage is the decision to move forward in spite of your fear.

Jesus was so deeply distressed and anguished by the suffering that awaited Him on the cross that "his sweat was like drops of blood falling to the ground" (Luke 22:44, NIV). This is a medically documented phenomenon known as hematidrosis, which is associated with fear and stress.

If you let it, fear can produce discouragement, depression, hopelessness, and paralysis. But fear can also motivate you to dig deep, stand strong, fight back, press on, and take massive action.

It's okay to feel afraid. There is no weakness in fear. Today I want to encourage you to be strong and channel your fear into positive, courageous action.

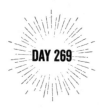

DAY 269

Every day of our lives, we are on the verge of making those slight changes that would make all the difference.

—Mignon McLaughlin

Don't underestimate those small changes, those little tweaks, that you can make to your routine, to your priorities, to your relationships, to your speech, and to your thoughts each day. Together, all of those small changes can make all the difference.

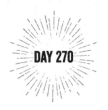

CALL SOMEONE YOU MISS TODAY

Life separates people. Sometimes for no particular reason. And you drift apart. And then, years go by.

Today, why don't you reconnect with someone you've lost touch with over the years? Your best friend from high school, your college roommate, a distant family member, your favorite coworker from two jobs ago . . .

Don't text. Call them on the phone and have a real conversation. Catch up. Tell them you miss them. Ask them about their life and their family.

Tell them how much you care about them and how much they mean to you. Tell them why you love them.

Reminisce and laugh about old times, strange teachers, crazy classmates, horrible bosses, the trouble you got into, the things you got away with . . . .

Encourage them if they are struggling.

Remind them how special they are.

Then ask them for money.

Just kidding.

Today's Challenge: *Call a special person from your past.*

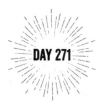

DAY 271

Love must be sincere. Hate what is evil; cling to what is good. Be devoted to one another in love. Honor one another above yourselves. Never be lacking in zeal, but keep your spiritual fervor, serving the Lord. Be joyful in hope, patient in affliction, faithful in prayer. Share with the Lord's people who are in need. Practice hospitality.

—Romans 12:9–13 (NIV)

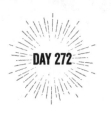

DAY 272

TRUTH IS SIMPLE.
LIES ARE COMPLICATED.

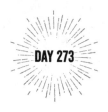

DAY 273

A heart at peace gives life to the body,
but envy rots the bones.

—Proverbs 14:30 (NIV)

Envy rots the bones? Yikes. That sounds pretty serious. Envy has always been a temptation for humans, but the widespread adoption of social media has created unprecedented levels of envy on a global scale. Never before in history have we been able to observe the lives of hundreds or thousands of people every day, many of whom try to present their life as perfect, glamorous, and enviable. But it's a lie. Everyone has problems. Don't be deceived. No one has a perfect life.

Envy steals contentment and stokes resentment. But a peaceful heart gives life to your body!

Today's Challenge: *Reduce envy. Reject envious thoughts when they creep in. If envy is a constant struggle, reduce your exposure and unfollow people who make you envious. And if you are trying to inspire envy in others with your social media posts, stop doing that.*

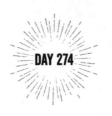

DAY 274

BECOME THE CURATOR OF LIFE. EDIT, LEAVE OUT THE JUNK. BUT WHEN YOU FIND SOMETHING WORTH KEEPING, TREASURE IT.

—ROBERT GREENE

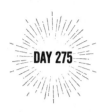

SUBTRACTION BEFORE ADDITION

When it comes to health and healing—solving problems and improving your quality of life—there are two things you need to think about: addition and subtraction.

Addition is asking, *What do I need to add to my life to make it better?* This is a good practice, but only thinking about adding things without thinking about what you need to subtract handicaps your problem-solving power and potential.

When I had cancer, I took ownership and responsibility for my situation. And I asked myself, "What do I need to eliminate from my life that could be contributing to my disease? What do I need to subtract? What needs to go?" I also prayed about it and said, "God, show me what I need to change." And then I took massive action to change my life.

I subtracted processed food, junk food, and animal-based food, and I added fruits and vegetables, fresh juices, and lots of supplements. I subtracted toxic cleaning and body-care products and replaced them with nontoxic brands. I looked at my thoughts and my attitudes and realized I needed to delete my bad habits, negative thinking, and unhealthy thought patterns and replace them with positivity, by choosing to be thankful and grateful instead of complaining and being negative, pessimistic, critical, and judgmental.

Addition without subtraction creates overwhelm. Subtraction makes room for addition.

Today's Question: *What can you subtract from your life to make it better?*

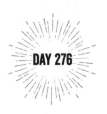

DAY 276

Brothers and sisters, whatever is true, whatever is noble, whatever is right, whatever is pure, whatever is lovely, whatever is admirable— if anything is excellent or praiseworthy—think about such things. Whatever you have learned or received or heard from me or seen in me—put it into practice. And the God of peace will be with you.

—Philippians 4:8–9 (NASB)

Remember: you can choose your thoughts. You can choose to dwell on things that cause you stress, anxiety, and fear— like your personal problems, other people's problems, all the problems happening around the world, and every worst-case scenario your imagination can conjure. Or you can choose to focus on things that bring you joy and happiness and gratitude. You can choose to think about all the good things you have, the people in your life who love you, and how much you have to be thankful for in spite of your circumstance. You can pay attention to people who encourage you and give you hope, joy, a new perspective, and fresh ideas.

You can marvel at the wisdom of God, who created an infinitely complex and perfectly ordered universe, and who created the earth for you! You can think about how amazing it is that your Heavenly Father cares about every detail of your life and that He loves you with an unfailing love and that He promised to give you peace, to supply all of your needs, and to never leave you or turn His back on you. Think about such things!

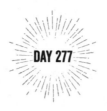

SLOTHS ARE CUTE, BUT DON'T BE ONE

The most underestimated factor that prevents a person from improving their life, their health, and their situation is laziness. Once upon a time, this state of being was known as sloth, for which my favorite definition is "a habitual disinclination to exertion."

Laziness is chronic lack of effort or making as little effort as possible. Laziness is a bad habit that over time becomes your modus operandi. Some people end up on lazy autopilot, always taking the laziest possible option. And the lazier you are, the more disorganized, chaotic, and unhealthy your life becomes. A hallmark of laziness is apathy and indifference, not caring about yourself or others. And let's not forget that sloth is one of the "seven deadly sins." It's the sin of not caring and not doing.

But laziness isn't genetic or terminal. Once you are mindful of your lazy tendencies, you can catch yourself in the act and say "I'm being lazy" and then bust through it by taking actions like making your bed, making juice, exercising, planning ahead, and keeping your house clean and organized. These actions will give you a sense of accomplishment and the energetic boost you need to do more and to resist your next lazy temptation.

Don't be lazy!

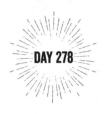

*If you do nothing in a difficult time,
your strength is limited.*

—Proverbs 24:10 (HCSB)

When things are difficult, it's easy to do nothing. And it's hard to get motivated when you are tired or discouraged or depressed or in pain.

There have been times in my life when I was struggling physically and emotionally, feeling sorry for myself, doing nothing, and praying that something would happen.

James 2:17 says that faith without works is dead.

Works is action! Faith plus action is a divine formula. When you take action, the strength and resources you need come to you. This is a universal principle.

Some days you have to force yourself to take action when you don't feel like it. You have to force yourself to make juice, to eat vegetables, to exercise when you have no energy . . . .

You may be telling yourself that you're not strong enough and that you're not ready to take action, but that's an excuse and a trap. Don't fall into it!

If you do nothing in a difficult time, your strength is limited.

But if you take action, your strength will increase!

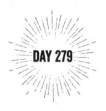

THE #2 CAUSE

Smoking is the #1 cause of cancer. Most of us know that. But the #2 cause of cancer is rarely discussed.

The second leading cause of cancer is obesity.

Excess body fat is a burden on your system. And being overweight is a disease state that promotes inflammation, reduces your immune function, and makes your body a place where cancer can thrive. That's not the kind of body you want.

Getting back to a healthy body weight, a normal body mass index (BMI), and getting rid of excess belly fat drops your risk of cancer recurrence and improves your odds of survival.

A whole-food, plant-based diet and daily aerobic exercise are the two most powerful and most sustainable weight loss promoters that work together in synergy. Periodic juice fasting and water fasting can also speed up the process.

Today is not about fat shaming. It is a loving reminder that your diet and lifestyle choices influence your health.

If you are overweight and cancer prevention and survival are priorities, now is the time to make a commitment to yourself to take massive action to get the excess weight off and make your body a lean, mean, cancer-fighting machine!

As always, make sure to consult your physician before making any significant dietary changes.

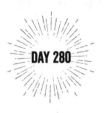

SERIOUSLY

You can radically change your diet and your lifestyle, exercise every day, and do every conventional and alternative therapy under the sun . . . but if you don't forgive the people who have hurt you and let go of your anger and bitterness toward them, you may not get well.

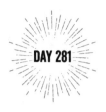

Look at the order in which you do things.

—BRIAN ENO AND PETER SCHMIDT, *OBLIQUE STRATEGIES*

Are you "out of order"? Perhaps your daily routine is out of order. Or your priorities are out of order. Can you rearrange your life and your schedule to be more efficient? More effective? Less stressful? I bet you can.

You are awake for 16 hours each day. You can accomplish a lot in 16 hours, if you are organized and disciplined.

Take a step back to reflect on the things you do each day—your good and bad habits—and the order in which you do these things. Where are you wasting time? (Hint: on your phone.)

Has taking care of yourself been a low priority? Spending time with your Heavenly Father, making healthy meals, juicing, exercise, and stress reduction need to be moved to the top of your priority list.

Take care of yourself so you can take care of others.

Your daily healing routine needs to be simple and sustainable. If it's too busy, difficult, and burdensome, you won't be able to keep it up.

Today's Challenge: *Look at the things you are doing and the order in which you are doing them.*

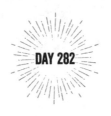

I HAVE TO DIE.
IF IT IS NOW, WELL THEN
I DIE NOW; IF LATER, THEN
NOW I WILL TAKE MY LUNCH,
SINCE THE HOUR FOR LUNCH
HAS ARRIVED—AND DYING
I WILL TEND TO LATER.

—EPICTETUS, *DISCOURSES*, BOOK 12

Making peace with death frees you to live your life without worry and fear.

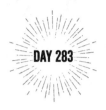

DON'T LOOK BACK

Forget the former things; do not dwell on the past. See, I am doing a new thing! Now it springs up; do you not perceive it? I am making a way in the wilderness and streams in the wasteland.

—Isaiah 43:18–19 (NIV)

Cancer divides your timeline into two sections: B.C. and A.D.—Before Cancer and After Diagnosis. The life you had before cancer is over. It's gone. You can't get it back.

When I was diagnosed with cancer, I grieved about losing the "carefree" life I had before. But I realized that I had to change in order to survive, so I let my old life go.

Seventeen years later, my A.D. life is so much better than my B.C. life was. Cancer put me on an entirely new path that I never imagined, and now I wouldn't trade my life for anything! That's the way I want you to look at your cancer situation. Don't look back, longing for the way things used to be. Look ahead, believing that God works all things for your good and that His plan is to prosper you and to give you abundant life.

Look ahead with the expectation that your future will be even better than your past. Your life will be better after cancer than it was before. Don't look back!

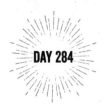

*You have a goal. And the action you take is either taking
you toward your goal or away from it. If your actions
take you away from your goal, that's self-sabotage.*

—Patti Digh, *Life Is a Verb*

We often think of self-sabotage as obviously destructive
actions—alcohol and drug abuse; self-harm; binge-eating;
picking fights; burning bridges; irresponsible, risky, and
dangerous behavior; and the like. And of course, all of those
things are. But self-sabotage also takes the form of seem-
ingly harmless and innocuous little choices each day that
prevent you from making progress toward your goals.

Excuses are a form of self-sabotage.

"It's no big deal" is a form of self-sabotage.

"I deserve a treat" is a form of self-sabotage.

"I don't feel like it" is a form of self-sabotage.

"I'll do it tomorrow" is a form of self-sabotage.

Once you become consciously aware of the big and little
ways you may be sabotaging your progress, you can catch
yourself in the act and foil the attempt.

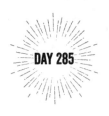

DAY 285

THE FEAR OF THE LORD LEADS TO LIFE, SO THAT ONE MAY SLEEP SATISFIED, UNTOUCHED BY EVIL.

—PROVERBS 19:23 (NASB)

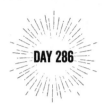

University of Alabama coach Nick Saban has a simple but powerful rule for his players: *be where your feet are*. Don't think about the last play or the next play. Instead, be in the moment and do exactly what you need to do right *now*! This is the mentality that wins football championships. And it's the mentality that you need to beat cancer.

On our journey back to health from Hodgkin's lymphoma, my wife, Cortney, and I had no idea what tomorrow would hold. But we knew that God is faithful, and that we could do our best with what He gave us each day. And so can you. You can research, read books, get a second opinion, change your diet, raise money, have conversations, extend forgiveness, embrace healing, love yourself, and enjoy today with faith, peace, and patience.

Focus on what He has placed in your hands and on your path at this moment. Do your very best with what you have, and trust that He will provide everything you need today.

Take a breath, scrunch up your toes, and feel the ground beneath you. *Be where your feet are.* This is where God's peace is found. And it's exactly where He has you.

—*Kevin Campbell*[36]

---

36 Kevin's wife, Cortney, was diagnosed with NLP Hodgkin's lymphoma in 2008 and healed with nutrition and nontoxic therapies. Learn more at www.anticancermom.com.

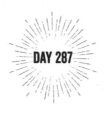

DAY 287

I DON'T FORGIVE PEOPLE BECAUSE I AM WEAK, I FORGIVE THEM BECAUSE I AM STRONG ENOUGH TO KNOW PEOPLE MAKE MISTAKES.

—UNKNOWN, ATTRIBUTED TO MARILYN MONROE

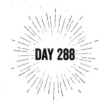

DO THE WORK

Transforming your health takes time and it takes work. You are changing your life and rebuilding your body. There is effort involved. No one else can do the work for you.

You have to do the work.

The work is not hard. You aren't digging ditches or breaking rocks on a chain gang.

The hardest part of this work is making the little choices each day, each moment, to do the things that move you closer to your goal. Even when you don't feel like it.

You have to choose to eat fruits and vegetables, not junk food. You have to choose to exercise when you don't want to. You have to choose to think positively and to count your blessings. You have to choose to make time to read the Bible, pray, meditate, and spend time with God, when you would rather stare at your phone or binge-watch TV shows.

This feels hard in the beginning because we don't like to change. But these are not hard things. This is easy work.

You have nothing to lose and everything to gain by taking care of yourself. Your quality of life and your survival depend on this work. You can do it.

So do the work.

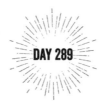

BEWARE THE SLIPPERY SLOPE

If you don't want to slip, don't go where it's slippery.

—Alcoholics Anonymous

As I've said before, 100 percent is easy; 99 percent is hard. That 1 percent difference is the slippery slope. Beware.

One hundred percent commitment is all the way. Ninety-nine percent gives you an out, an excuse, a little wiggle room.

You skip another day of exercise. You go through the drive-thru. You buy junk food at the grocery store "for other people." You prioritize unimportant things. You withhold forgiveness. You tell yourself you don't have enough time. You look for opinions that give you permission to not do what you need to do. You distance yourself from people who love you and are trying to hold you accountable.

The little 1 percent—the exception, the permission to quit, to slack off, to backslide, to self-sabotage—can easily grow to 2 percent, then 5 percent, then 10 percent, then 20 percent without your even noticing. And somewhere along the way, your progress slows down, then stops, and then you start going downhill and your plan falls apart. And further down the slope you slide. And then you find yourself at the bottom, with no idea how it happened.

The slippery slope is easy to get on, but it's also easy to get off. If you catch yourself slipping, get off the slippery slope!

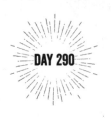

THE NAME OF THE LORD IS A STRONG TOWER; THE RIGHTEOUS RUNS INTO IT AND IS SAFE.

—PROVERBS 18:10 (NASB)

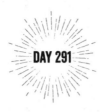

THINGS ASTRONAUT CHRIS HADFIELD TAUGHT ME

Lack of knowledge, lack of preparation, and your imagination running wild with worst-case scenarios for an unknown future all create fear. The more you know, the less you fear.

Things aren't scary. People are scared.

It makes sense to feel fear when you are in danger. That's rational fear. But many people choose to be afraid of all kinds of things that are not dangerous, that have not even happened or are not likely to happen. That's irrational fear.

If you say, "I'm going to take a risk because it's worth it," that changes your part.

You are no longer a spectator or a passenger. You are taking an active role to minimize your risk of harm or danger, in order to solve a problem or accomplish a meaningful goal.

Ask yourself:

- *What are the risks worth taking?*
- *If they do make me afraid, why?*

Then identify the actions you can take to reduce your risk and your fear. And take them.

The best antidote for fear is competence.[37]

---

37 Editor's note: This excerpt is from the Chris Hadfield MasterClass.

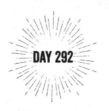

RAISE YOUR STANDARDS

You have permission to do anything you want and to eat anything you want. And you always will. No one is taking away your favorite foods. But if your favorite foods or habits are harmful to your health, your standards are too low.

The pursuit of health isn't about what you can't do; it's about what you can do. Unhealthy choices should not be viewed as forbidden, but rather as things you don't want to do. Things you choose not to do.

Those things are beneath you now because you've raised your standards.

You are worthy of the highest standards. Your mind, body, and spirit deserve the utmost love and care because you are a child of God. Your Heavenly Father loves you with an everlasting love.

Your body is a temple of the Holy Spirit. And you are the caretaker. Give your body the highest-quality whole foods from the earth. Give your body invigorating exercise six days a week. Give your body eight hours of rest each night. Take every thought captive. Don't worry about the future. Give your worries and fears to the Lord. Fix your eyes on Jesus, the author and perfecter of your faith.

Raise your standards.

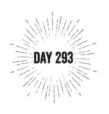

LUCK IS NOT A FACTOR.
HOPE IS NOT A STRATEGY.
FEAR IS NOT AN OPTION.

—JAMES CAMERON

There are reasons people survive or don't survive cancer, and they have nothing to do with how lucky or unlucky they are. Luck is not a factor.

Hope and faith must be infused with action. Hope alone is not a strategy.

Fear paralyzes you, pollutes your intelligence, and steals your joy. Fear is not an option.

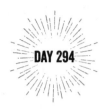

DAY 294

Whether you believe you can do a thing or not, you are right.

—OFTEN ATTRIBUTED TO HENRY FORD

Henry Ford did things which had never been done before—monumental, world-changing things. And just like countless other successful people throughout history, Henry Ford was driven by the belief that he could achieve great things. You must believe that about yourself now. Stop doubting yourself and stop talking yourself out of taking action with those two little words . . . "I can't."

"I can't" cripples you. Stop saying it.

If you don't want to do something, say "I don't want to."

Replace "I can't do this" with "I can do this." And if you aren't sure how, ask yourself, "How can I do this?" That's how you turn on your creative problem-solving brain! And that's where the process of discovery begins.

Even if no one else believes in you. Even if everyone tells you "You can't." You must believe in yourself. And you must believe that you can because you have the love and unlimited resources of your Heavenly Father, the Creator of the universe, at your disposal. You can do all things through Him who gives you strength (Philippians 4:13)!

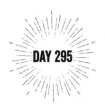

DAY 295

Now to Him who is able to do far more abundantly beyond all that we ask or think, according to the power that works within us, to Him be the glory in the church and in Christ Jesus to all generations forever and ever. Amen.

—Ephesians 3:20 (NASB)

Is your problem too complicated? Are your needs too great? Is your dream too big? No!

Exercise your faith and believe that your Heavenly Father, who loves you, can do abundantly beyond all that you can ask or imagine! Because His power is at work in you.

Choose to believe big and start asking for big things: the biggest, most impossible things you can imagine. Let gigantic dreams well up in your heart and ask for them to be accomplished. And expect that He will do more than you ask or even think is even possible!

Burn this into your brain. Plaster it on the wall. Confess it out of your mouth. Pray it often.

Father, thank you that you are able to do far more abundantly beyond all that I ask or think, according to your power that works in me!

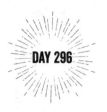

FOLLOW THE LEADER

It's easy to be a follower. To never have to make hard decisions. To go with the flow. To just do what other people tell you to do. Maybe you've always been a follower. Maybe you've never felt like or wanted to be a leader. . . .

The truth is that you are a leader. You are the leader of your thoughts and actions. You are the leader of every cell in your body. Every day you are leading them toward health or disease with your choices.

Great leaders don't have all the experience or expertise or all the answers. But great leaders always have these qualities: They have a clear vision of where they want to go. And they have focus—the ability to ignore all the noise and distractions and anything that doesn't move them toward their goals. Great leaders know they can't accomplish big things alone. They surround themselves with smart people to advise them. And they are decisive. Great leaders know when to keep going and when to change course. Now more than ever, you must become the leader that God created you to be. You must lead yourself. Don't be afraid. You are not alone. Make a plan, follow the plan, and trust that the Lord will direct your steps (Proverbs 16:9).

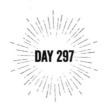

In his first letter to the early churches, the Apostle John talks about asking and receiving from God:

> *Dear friends, if our hearts do not condemn us, we have confidence before God and receive from Him anything we ask, because we keep his commands and do what pleases him.*
> —1 John 3:21–22 (NIV)

> *These things I have written to you who believe in the name of the Son of God, so that you may know that you have eternal life. This is the confidence which we have before Him, that, if we ask anything according to His will, He hears us. And if we know that He hears us in whatever we ask, we know that we have the requests which we have asked from Him.*
> —1 John 5:13–15 (NASB)

If your heart is in the right place—your conscience is clean and you are not living in disobedience (by not forgiving those who've hurt you, for example)—you can approach your Heavenly Father with the confidence that He will give you whatever you ask for, according to His will.

This is where your faith must be exercised. You must believe that it is God's will to heal you and that He will grant your request.

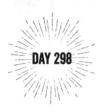

DAY 298

There's an old joke in Christian circles: "Never pray for patience." Because that's basically asking God to put you into an unpleasant situation that forces you to be patient, and you are not going to enjoy it.

Being impatient isn't just about being in a rush or hurry. Impatience is rooted in selfishness, a lack of love and kindness, and even a lack of faith in God's perfect timing.

Patience is a fruit of the Holy Spirit (Galatians 4:22).

Patience is an act of love, because love is patient and kind (1 Corinthians 13:4).

Our Heavenly Father loves us with an everlasting love, and He wants us to be patient like Him. His love, kindness, and patience with us are infinite and incalculable!

Patience isn't something you need to pray for. It's something you need to practice.

A simple prayer of patience:

Father, thank you for giving me patience and peace. I will be patient in my circumstance, trusting that You will supply all of my needs and work all things for my good. I will wait upon You to renew my strength. I choose to be patient, loving, and kind to myself and others today.

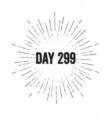

THE PEOPLE YOU MOST WANT TO HELP ARE USUALLY THE PEOPLE YOU CANNOT HELP.

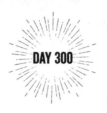

DAY 300

HE'S GOT THIS

God uses every circumstance we go through in life to show us His strength and power. I know you've heard people say, "God won't give you anything you can't handle." But I believe He often allows us to go through situations that are too much for us to handle *by ourselves*. During these hard times, we learn how much we need Him. And we learn to trust and rely on the One who created us and loves us with an infinite everlasting love.

Hebrews 11:1 (NIV) says, "Faith is confidence in what we hope for and assurance about what we do not see." In difficult times, it's important for you to remember to focus on the capability of God instead of the challenge before you. Each day you have a choice to make. Will you give in to the fear, or will you live by faith and fight? How do I do this? I remind myself that God did not give me a spirit of fear, but one of power, love, and a sound mind. I remember that He promised me that He would never fail me or leave me. And that He promises to be faithful, *even* when I am all but out of faith.

Remember today that courage is not being fearless, but the ability to act in the face of fear. Take the step to Believe God for big things in your life because He turns our adversity into victory, our obstacles into opportunities, and our problems into possibilities.

—Ivelisse Page, founder of Believe Big and survivor of stage IV colon cancer[38]

---

38 Connect with Ivelisse Page at www.believebig.org.

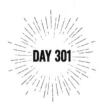

DAY 301

To live is the rarest thing in the world.
Most people exist, that is all.

—Oscar Wilde

Death is not a choice. You cannot choose whether or not to die. Because death is inevitable for all of us. Like it or not, it's coming.

Accepting and making peace with death gives you the freedom to live without fear.

And in the meantime, between this moment and your last breath, whenever that may be, you can choose life. You can choose to live your life to the fullest, like you never have before.

You can choose how to live, where to live, and why to live.

Or you can choose to just exist—taking up space, consuming air, water, food, and media, doing nothing, and providing no value to the world while you wait for your eventual demise.

Every day you have choices to make. And your choices have a profound influence on how long you live and the quality of your life. You can't stop death, but you can slow it down!

So today is just another loving reminder from me that your choices matter, the big ones and the little ones.

Choose to live today!

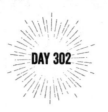

DAY 302

I consider it an error to trust and hope in any means or efforts in themselves alone; nor do I consider it a safe path to trust the whole matter to God our Lord without desiring to help myself by what he has given me; so that it seems to me in our Lord that I ought to make use of both parts, desiring in all things his greater praise and glory, and nothing else.

—St. Ignatius of Loyola

In other words, pray as if everything depends on God and work as if everything depends on you.

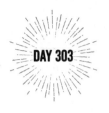

DAY 303

The impediment to action advances action.
What stands in the way becomes the way.

—Marcus Aurelius, *Meditation*

Impediments, barricades, obstacles, challenges, and opposition are normal parts of life and parts of every journey. They often come as a surprise, but don't be discouraged, depressed, or stressed by them. They are necessary. Obstacles make your journey uniquely yours. They test you, stretch you, and teach you. Obstacles are a good thing. They make you smarter and stronger. They are a blessing in disguise. Be thankful for obstacles and that your Heavenly Father will guide you through them.

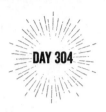

BE PERSISTENT IN PRAYER

Jesus said to his disciples, "Suppose one of you has a friend, and goes to him at midnight and says to him, 'Friend, lend me three loaves; for a friend of mine has come to me from a journey, and I have nothing to set before him'; and from inside he answers and says, 'Do not bother me; the door has already been shut and my children and I are in bed; I cannot get up and give you anything.'

"I tell you, even though he will not get up and give him anything because he is his friend, yet because of his persistence he will get up and give him as much as he needs.

"So I say to you, ask, and it will be given to you; seek, and you will find; knock, and it will be opened to you. For everyone who asks, receives; and he who seeks, finds; and to him who knocks, it will be opened."

—Luke 11:5–10 (NASB)

Jesus told this parable to explain the way you need to pray. Be persistent. Keep asking God for what you want and for what you need. Keep asking. Keep seeking. Keep knocking on the door. Don't let up until you get it.

Are you bothering God? Maybe. But Jesus told the parable. So, it's okay to do it!

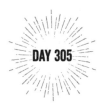

LOVE YOUR BODY

I had a weird body growing up. I was a shrimpy little kid, one of the shortest and skinniest in my class. I got made fun of, and I became extremely insecure about it. In high school, I shot up to six-feet-two and became one of the tallest in my class. But I didn't fill out like everyone else. I was still unusually thin, and I wore baggy clothes to hide it. To me, being the skinny kid was embarrassing and shameful. I hated my body. I saw myself as inferior and flawed. I wanted so badly to be "normal," and I was jealous and resented other guys who were physically superior. In college, my insecurity motivated me to work out and I gained some weight. I felt like I looked better, but my insecurity remained.

After my diagnosis, I began to wonder if cancer was my body's way of rebelling against me for hating it for so many years. Maybe my toxic, insecure thoughts had weakened my immune system and created an environment where cancer could thrive. . . .

So I made a decision to stop hating my body, and I chose to love it. I loved my body with what I put in it, what I put on it, and how I treated it with exercise and rest. I even started thinking to myself, *I love my body*. I started thanking God for my body. And I looked in the mirror and told myself, *I love you*.

If you've been hating on your body, today's challenge is to love on it. Capture those toxic, insecure thoughts when they creep in and kick them out of your mind. Show your body love by choosing to take care of it. And look in the mirror and tell your body, *I love you. Let's get better.*

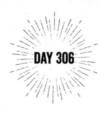

DAY 306

I love the Lord, because He hears
My voice and *my supplications.*

Because He has inclined His ear to me,
Therefore I shall call upon Him *as long as I live.*

The cords of death encompassed me
And the terrors of Sheol (hell) came upon me;
I found distress and sorrow.

Then I called upon the name of the Lord:
"O Lord, I beseech You, save my life!"

Gracious is the Lord, and righteous;
Yes, our God is compassionate.

The Lord preserves the simple;
I was brought low, and He saved me.

Return to your rest, O my soul,
For the Lord has dealt bountifully with you.

For You have rescued my soul from death,
My eyes from tears, my feet from stumbling.

I shall walk before the Lord
In the land of the living.

—Psalm 116:1–9 (NASB)

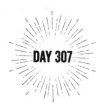

GET OFF AUTOPILOT

We are living, breathing computers, and over time we become programmed. We get stuck in patterns of thought and behavior, and most of our days we operate like robots.

The food you eat. The way you think. Judgmental thoughts. Insecure thoughts. Negative self-talk. The things you get upset about. Your grooming habits. Your exercise routine, or lack thereof. The way you work. The time you spend on social media or zoned out in front of the TV. The way you treat the people in your life. The way you interact with strangers. The way you deal with stress.

Negative patterns will eventually produce problems in your life. If your life is a chaotic mess, your autopilot may be inadvertently set to self-destruct mode.

Radical life change means getting off autopilot. You need pattern interruption. You need to deliberately break your normal routine, even if you like your normal routine.

Eat fruits and vegetables. Go to work a different way. Exercise when you don't feel like it. Reject negative and critical thoughts. Bite your tongue. Stop gossiping. Take an extended break from social media. Read a book instead of watching TV. Treat everyone in your life better.

As you consistently replace negative patterns with positive ones, you reprogram yourself, and eventually your new autopilot will be one that continually and effortlessly promotes health and healing.

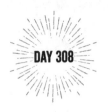

MIRACLE INTERFERENCE

Jesus left there and went to his hometown, accompanied by his disciples. When the Sabbath came, He began to teach in the synagogue, and many who heard Him were amazed.

"Where did this man get these things?" they asked. "What's this wisdom that has been given him? What are these remarkable miracles he is performing? Isn't this the carpenter? Isn't this Mary's son and the brother of James, Joseph, Judas and Simon? Aren't his sisters here with us?" And they took offense at him.

Jesus said to them, "A prophet is not without honor except in his own town, among his relatives and in his own home." He could not do any miracles there, except lay his hands on a few sick people and heal them. He was amazed at their lack of faith.

—Mark 6:1–6 (NIV)

In this instance, the unbelief of the people around Jesus was so strong that His ability to perform miracles and heal the sick was hindered; it was blocked by unbelief. If you are surrounded by people with no faith for healing—your family, your friends, even your church—it could be interfering with the process. Find a church—a community of believers—that has faith for miraculous healing and sees it happen regularly. There are churches like this in every city. Align yourself with faith-filled prayer warriors who will lay hands on you and pray for you to be healed.

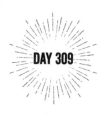

THOSE WHO THINK THEY HAVE NOT TIME FOR BODILY EXERCISE WILL SOONER OR LATER HAVE TO FIND TIME FOR ILLNESS.

—EDWARD STANLEY, EARL OF DERBY

The Earl of Derby was onto something. A four-year study published in 2020 that followed over 8,000 people found that those who were the most sedentary, or spent the most time sitting, had a 52 percent increased risk of death from cancer compared to the most active people.[39]

So get moving! You need at least 150 minutes of exercise per week. That's 25 minutes per day six days per week. Find time for exercise today.

---

39 Gilchrist et al., "Association of Sedentary Behavior With Cancer Mortality in Middle-Aged and Older US Adults," *JAMA Oncology* (June 18, 2020): e202045. doi:10.1001/jamaoncol.2020.2045.

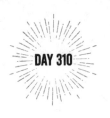

DAY 310

INACTION BREEDS DOUBT AND FEAR. ACTION BREEDS CONFIDENCE AND COURAGE. IF YOU WANT TO CONQUER FEAR, DO NOT SIT HOME AND THINK ABOUT IT. GO OUT AND GET BUSY.

—OFTEN ATTRIBUTED TO DALE CARNEGIE

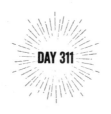

WATCH THIS

Today is another reminder to stop watching the news and dramas and stress-inducing shows and instead watch shows that dose you with laughter and joy, like comedies. One really fun show that I recommend is *America's Got Talent*.

You will laugh.

You will cry.

And you will be touched by the stories and amazed by the perseverance, triumph, and incredible talent of your fellow humans, from children all the way to senior citizens. There are singers, dancers, acrobats, daredevils, comedians, magicians, and people with talents you can't even imagine.

America's Got Talent will bring you so much joy and inspiration. And you need that in your life in megadoses.

There are 15 seasons of *AGT* to date. That will keep you entertained and inspired for a long time.

And who knows? Maybe I'll see you on that stage one day, superstar!

P.S. *America's Got Talent* did not pay me to promote their show.

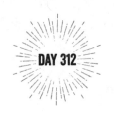

DAY 312

**EVERY DAY IS A
NEW BEGINNING.**

**DON'T LET YESTERDAY'S
MISTAKES INFLUENCE
TODAY'S ATTITUDE
OR ACTIONS.**

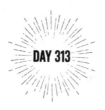

DAY 313

The key to growth is to learn to make promises and to keep them.

—Stephen R. Covey

Keep your promises. Honor your commitments. Be a person of your word. Do what you say you are going to do.

Generally speaking, we're pretty good at keeping the promises we make to others because we don't want to disappoint them and/or hurt our reputation.

The hardest promises to keep are the ones we make to ourselves.

When you continually break your promises to yourself or others, guilt and shame creep in and you end up liking yourself less and less. Forgive yourself and start fresh.

Now is the time to make a promise to yourself to radically change your life. To break your bad habits. To take care of yourself every day in a way that you never have before. To make a healing plan and stick with it. To fight fear and doubt with faith. To forgive those who have hurt you. To trust in the Lord with all of your heart.

Keep the promises you make to yourself.

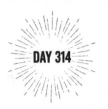

THAT OTHER REASON TO FORGIVE

I've talked about the importance of forgiveness a lot, and I've given you many different reasons to forgive throughout this book.

But if you are still holding out on forgiving some people in your life, here's something else to consider:

Jesus said, "If you forgive other people when they sin against you, your heavenly Father will also forgive you. But if you do not forgive others their sins, your Father will not forgive your sins" (Matthew 6:14–15, NIV).

According to Jesus, unforgiveness has eternal consequences, which will follow you beyond the grave.

That's the scariest reason of all to not forgive.

So let's not take any chances. The stakes are way too high.

Today is the day to forgive. Stop putting it off.

Choose to forgive those who have hurt you right now. Let them go. Give them to God. Ask Him to bless them. And let Him deal with them. And thank Him for forgiving you.

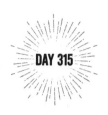

DAY 315

COURAGE IS LIKE—IT'S A HABITUS, A HABIT, A VIRTUE: YOU GET IT BY COURAGEOUS ACTS. IT'S LIKE YOU LEARN TO SWIM BY SWIMMING. YOU LEARN COURAGE BY COURAGING.

—MARIE MAYNARD DALY, PH.D.[40]

---

40 Dr. Marie Maynard Daly was the first African American woman to receive a doctorate in chemistry in the United States.

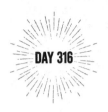

DO I HAVE YOUR ATTENTION?

God used cancer to get my attention. He wanted me to turn to Him and trust Him fully. I needed to get to the point where He was sufficient. My health and my marriage were in shambles, but cancer taught me to trust that He was going to use it all for my good. There are no mistakes in God's plans; He had me exactly where He wanted me.

Trials help us grow more reliant on God. They help us grow in faith. They help us realize that while we are powerless and weak, God is powerful, faithful, and sovereign. He is in control of every aspect of our lives—the good, the bad, and the ugly.

In the midst of the storm, we must trust our Creator. Fretting and worrying aren't trusting. Worry is rooted in a belief that He is not enough. He is. Your walk will not be perfect, but stay in the Word, guard your heart, and renew your mind each day. This is essential to help you navigate the toughest times of your life.

Even though I would never have chosen this path, I am thankful for the growth and blessings that have come from my cancer journey (Philippians 4:4–9).

—*Julie Johnson, breast cancer survivor*

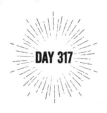

ALL THE DAYS OF THE AFFLICTED ARE BAD, BUT A CHEERFUL HEART HAS A CONTINUAL FEAST.

—PROVERBS 15:15 (NASB)

The state of affliction and a cheerful heart are both choices.

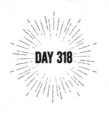

DAY 318

Delight yourself in the Lord;
And He will give you the desires of your heart.
Commit your way to the Lord,
Trust also in Him, and He will do it.
He will bring forth your righteousness as the light
and your judgment as the noonday.

Rest in the Lord and wait patiently for Him;
Do not fret because of him who prospers in his way,
Because of the man who carries out wicked schemes.
Cease from anger and forsake wrath;
Do not fret; it leads only to evildoing.

—Psalm 37:4–8 (NASB)

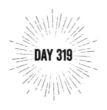

FLY YOUR FAILURE FLAG HIGH

Never be afraid to expose a weakness in yourself.
Exposing a weakness is the beginning of strength.

—ROBERT ANTHONY, *BEYOND POSITIVE THINKING*

So you've made some bad decisions. You've made some mistakes . . . stupid, selfish mistakes. And you are embarrassed and ashamed. And you hope no one finds out. And you beat yourself up. And maybe you don't feel worthy of a good life, success, health, love, happiness, or forgiveness.

Here's a new strategy. Let your secrets out. Hold your failures up like a banner for the world to see.

Your mistakes taught you powerful lessons that you need to pass on. Sharing your painful, embarrassing mistakes can change lives or even save lives, but not if you keep them a secret.

You can use your failures for good! Sharing your story can prevent others from making the same painful mistakes. And using your failures and mistakes to help others frees you from the pain and shame you've been carrying.

You have a unique and beautiful story, mistakes and all. The world needs you to share it.

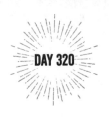

DAY 320

THE REWARD OF HUMILITY AND THE FEAR OF THE LORD ARE RICHES, HONOR, AND LIFE.

—PROVERBS 22:4 (NASB)

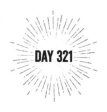

ON YOUR OWN TERMS

Once you reach adulthood, no one is responsible for your life but you. You have to live with the choices you make. You reap the rewards of good choices and you suffer the consequences of bad ones. And of course, your choices also affect the people around you.

No one can live your life for you, and ultimately no one should dictate the direction of your life.

Cancer is a disease that requires difficult decisions. People around you are going to try to help you and save you. Now, more than ever, you must be up-front and honest with your doctors and loved ones. Tell them exactly what you want and what you don't want.

Don't let anyone rush you into doing something you don't want to do out of fear or peer pressure.

You should not risk your life or suffer needlessly to appease your doctors or the people around you who don't understand what you really want just because you are afraid to say no.

This is your life. You should live and die on your own terms, not according to someone else's plan, schedule, or timeline.

Live and die on your own terms.

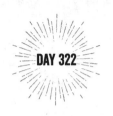

DAY 322

WHEN JESUS LANDED AND SAW A LARGE CROWD, HE HAD COMPASSION ON THEM AND HEALED THEIR SICK.

—MATTHEW 14:14 (NIV)

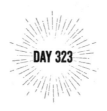

I had no intention of starting a blog or making videos or writing books when I had cancer. But I did have a sense that God would use it in some way. Six and a half years after my diagnosis, I started chrisbeatcancer.com to give hope and encouragement to cancer patients, caregivers, and health-conscious folks. And just as a tiny seed can grow into a huge tree over time, God multiplied my effort exponentially.

Do you have a big vision? Do you want to make an impact in the world? Do you want to leave a legacy of love and service and lives changed? I hope so. If this resonates, I have two pieces of advice for you.

First, start thinking and dreaming and praying about what you want to do in the future, right now. No dream or idea is too big. Write your vision and ideas down. The time to start is when you can't stand waiting any longer.

Second, no matter how much good you do, there will always be those who think you're doing it wrong, you aren't doing enough, or you're doing it for the wrong reasons. Some people may even maliciously twist things you say and do to make you look bad.

The more impact you have, the fiercer your opponents get. Criticism is painful. But it is necessary. It sharpens you and toughens you up. Expect it, but don't waste your time and energy on the critics. You have more important work to do.

Just keep doing good!

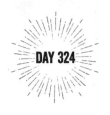

A THANKFUL HEART IS NOT ONLY THE GREATEST VIRTUE, BUT THE PARENT OF ALL THE OTHER VIRTUES.

—CICERO

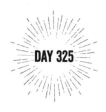

TAKE EVERY THOUGHT CAPTIVE

We control our thoughts, and our thoughts influence our emotions. Negative thoughts produce negative, harmful emotions. And when our emotions run wild, we think irrational, unhealthy, destructive thoughts. It can be a vicious cycle.

If you let your emotions rule, you will make impulsive, irrational decisions that create chaos, unhappiness, and disease in your life.

When negative thoughts, anxiety, and fear creep in to sabotage your happiness and peace of mind, you have to catch them. Pounce on them, take them captive, tie them up, and throw them out!

It doesn't always come easy, but remember: you have the power to choose to think positively and to look for the silver lining in every situation.

The most powerful thoughts are those of gratitude. Counting your blessings will reset your perspective and crowd out the negative thoughts and emotions with thankfulness, peace, and joy.

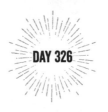

SWITCH FILTERS

Your mind has a filter through which all information passes. This filter is shaped by your education and life experiences, and it informs your opinions, emotions, and decisions. And over time, one of two polarities tends to become more dominant: positive or negative.

The negative filter finds faults and flaws in every person and situation. And the practice of negative filtering makes you increasingly more insecure, critical, cynical, skeptical, pessimistic, and unhappy. That was the pattern I was stuck in before cancer.

But cancer taught me that I was in control of my filter and that I could swap it out in an instant. In any situation I could choose to look for the positive, the bright side, and the silver lining instead of focusing on the negative. And you can too!

A positive filter is full of faith, open to new ideas, hopeful, optimistic, resourceful, nonjudgmental, loving, and forgiving, and it chooses to believe the best about people.

Today's Challenge: *When you catch yourself having negative thoughts, visualize turning a dial in your head to switch your filter from negative to positive with a click. And then use your positive filter to reassess the situation. Eventually the positive filter will become your default.*

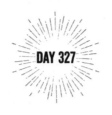

DAY 327

EVERY CELL IN YOUR BODY IS EAVESDROPPING ON YOUR THOUGHTS.

—DEEPAK CHOPRA

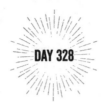

DAY 328

WIN THE MORNING, WIN THE DAY

How you start your morning can set the tone for your entire day. Here are some suggestions to help you create a more peaceful and productive morning routine.

Start your morning with gratitude. Thank God for another day of life and for everything else you can think of. Then make your bed.

Don't check your phone. Don't even touch your phone. Don't get on your computer. Don't turn on the TV. Avoid all news.

Go outside. Go for a walk, or a run, or do whatever kind of exercise you like. Tend to your garden.

Make juice or tea.

Spend a few minutes reading the Bible. Spend a few minutes in prayer. Spend a few minutes meditating, focusing on your breath.

Journal. Write down three things you are thankful for. Write down your thoughts, your prayer requests, your affirmations, and your three highest priorities for the day.

Hug and kiss your loved ones. Tell them you how much you love them and why. And tell yourself, *Today is going to be a great day!*

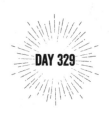

THE MIND OF MAN PLANS HIS WAY, BUT THE LORD DIRECTS HIS STEPS.

—PROVERBS 16:9 (NASB)

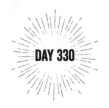

HARMONIZE WITH ME

Most illness is just stress from not living in harmony.

—Bruce Lipton

Health is a natural by-product of living in harmony with nature. But unfortunately, we have gotten really far away from harmonious living. Think about every aspect of your life: your daily habits, what you eat, how you spend your time, where you live, where you work, the type of work you do, where you sleep, when you sleep . . . .

It's shocking how little our daily lives have in common with the daily lives of our ancestors. They spent most of their time outside, doing physical work, getting lots of fresh air and sunshine, walking everywhere, growing and eating their own whole, unprocessed food (mostly plants), not watching television, not on the Internet, blissfully ignorant of world events, and going to bed within a few hours of sundown, to name a few things.

Fortunately, you don't have to travel back to biblical times to incorporate many of the things I listed above into your daily life.

Today's Challenge: *Ask yourself the question I asked myself back in 2004: How can I live in a way that is more in harmony with nature?*

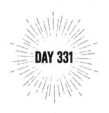

SERVE

Cancer is a unique season of your life. Self-care must become a priority, but if you obsess over yourself and cancer too much, it can be counterproductive and stressful and make you bonkers.

You need balance. And you need to get out of your own head.

Serving others is a form of self-care. Look for new and unique ways to serve people outside of your normal obligations, without expecting anything in return or committing yourself to anything that could add stress to your life. Volunteer to serve at an event at your church, a children's hospital, a nursing home, a homeless shelter, or any other charity. Give your time to help and serve others, but without making their problems your problems.

Is there someone you can mentor or minister to, give helpful advice, recommend for a promotion? Do you know someone who is elderly, widowed, a single parent, or disabled who needs their dog walked, or their yard cut, or their car washed, or help with errands, or a meal, or just a friendly visit?

Serving others is therapeutic. It gets your mind off yourself and your situation. It gives you joy, fulfillment, satisfaction, and a new sense of purpose. It's good for them and it's good for you.

Today's Challenge: *Look for people and opportunities to serve.*

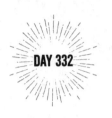

DAY 332

THE BLIND AND THE LAME CAME TO HIM IN THE TEMPLE, AND HE [JESUS] HEALED THEM.

—MATTHEW 21:14 (NIV)

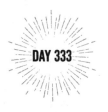

DON'T DEFER YOUR HAPPINESS

Internet fame, a large following, and a best-selling book did not add a single ounce of happiness to my life . . . because I was already happy. Cancer taught me how to be happy in the most difficult season of my life. It taught me that happiness comes from inside, not from accomplishments and stuff.

It's okay to have dreams and desires to be more, to do more, to have more. It's okay to work to create a better life for yourself. You should! But don't defer your happiness into the future. Don't fall into the happier future trap. *I'll be happy when X happens. . . . I'll be happy when I have more money . . . when I get a better job . . . when I'm cancer free . . . .*

If you aren't happy without the things you want, you won't be happy after you get them. You will eventually be less happy! And if you aren't thankful and content with what you have right now, why should you expect God to bless you with more?

If your happiness is contingent on other people or circumstances, you will continue to be disappointed, frustrated, and unhappy.

Gratitude is the secret to happiness and contentment. And if you figure out how to be happy now, you'll also be happy later when you get the things that you're dreaming about, praying for, and working toward. Your happiness is up to you. Be happy now!

WRESTLEMANIA

Do you need help? Do you need healing? Do you need peace? Do you need encouragement? Do you need joy?

Then you need to pray.

There isn't anyone you need to talk to more than God.

In Genesis 32:22–32, it says that Jacob wrestled with God all night and would not let go until God blessed him. And He did!

Jesus said, "When you pray, go into your inner room, close your door and pray to your Father who is in secret, and your Father who sees *what is done* in secret will reward you" (Matthew 6:6, NASB).

Jesus also said, "Ask, and it will be given to you" (Matthew 7:7, NASB) and "If you believe, you will receive whatever you ask for in prayer" (Matthew 21:22, NIV).

Pray passionately. Pray fervently. Pray continually. Every day throughout the day. Cry out to God, your Heavenly Father, who cares about every detail of your life.

Fight for your life. Wrestle with God like Jacob did. Don't let go until you get what you need. And believe that you will.

Believe that you will see your prayers answered and that miracles will happen in your life!

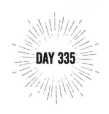

DAY 335

CONTROL WHAT YOU CAN CONTROL—YOUR THOUGHTS, YOUR WORDS, AND YOUR ACTIONS—AND GIVE THE REST TO GOD.

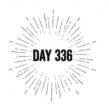

ZOOM OUT

Think of your mind as a camera with interchangeable lenses. These lenses change the way you interpret people, your circumstances, and everything around you.

A macro lens lets you zoom in super close to focus on the tiniest details, like an ant carrying a leaf down a bamboo shoot. A wide-angle lens lets you zoom way out to see the whole scene, a vast forest in the foothills of a mountain range under a cloudy sky.

If you zoom in too close, you lose context. If you zoom out too far, you lose detail.

Sometimes you need to zoom in on the details in order to gain more understanding. At other times you need to zoom out to get proper perspective so you can see the big picture.

Both lenses are necessary, but too often we get stuck zoomed in. We "miss the forest for the trees," and we blow minor problems way out of proportion.

Today's Challenge: *Zoom out. Pop on your wide-angle lens and look at your daily concerns in the broader context of your whole life and eternity. Ask yourself,* Will this problem matter tomorrow, next week, next month, or next year? *And let the answer reset your perspective.*

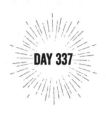

TO MAKE MISTAKES IS HUMAN.
TO OWN YOUR MISTAKES IS DIVINE.
NOTHING ELEVATES A PERSON HIGHER
THAN QUICKLY ADMITTING AND TAKING
PERSONAL RESPONSIBILITY FOR THE
MISTAKES YOU MAKE AND THEN FIXING
THEM FAIRLY. IF YOU MESS UP, FESS
UP. IT'S ASTOUNDING HOW POWERFUL
THIS OWNERSHIP IS.

—KEVIN KELLY

GET A MASSAGE

Let people touch you and work on your physical body.

Get massage therapy, chiropractic adjustments, structural integration (aka Rolfing), acupuncture, or all of the above several times per week, or as much as you are able.

Bodywork therapies can reduce your stress, improve your mood, increase blood and lymphatic fluid circulation, accelerate detoxification, and even enhance your immune function.

You need this, and you deserve it. But there's also another reason. . . .

You need to spend time with healers.

Practitioners of the healing arts can be invaluable sources of encouragement, resources, and information. They are connectors. They know things you need to know. And they know people you need to know.

Tell them who you are. Tell them your story. Ask them what they would do if they were you. And ask them who they think you should go see.

And then go see those people. Adventure awaits . . .

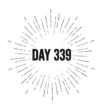

DON'T CHASE SHINY OBJECTS

Throughout life, and especially on a healing journey, there are countless shiny objects vying for your attention. Every new discovery you make appears better than what you are doing. It may be a different dietary strategy or a new supplement or a new treatment. . . . I've seen many patients with "shiny object syndrome" constantly jumping from one thing to the next, trying to get well but never getting there because they weren't disciplined enough to stick with anything long enough to know if it helped them.

There are a lot of treatment options and healing strategies out there. And you can't do them all. You have to choose something and get started. That's your Plan A. Make your plan, work your plan, and measure your results along the way—every 30, 60, or 90 days. Expect to make adjustments along the way, but don't change course and jump to Plan B until you are certain that Plan A isn't helping you.

You must be diligent, disciplined, and methodical. If you don't track your changes and monitor your progress, you will waste precious time and money and reduce your odds of success. Don't chase shiny objects.

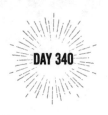

DAY 340

*Some became fools through their rebellious ways
and suffered affliction because of their iniquities.
They loathed all food
and drew near the gates of death.
Then they cried to the Lord in their trouble,
and he saved them from their distress.
He sent out his word and healed them;
he rescued them from the grave.
Let them give thanks to the Lord for his unfailing love
and his wonderful deeds for mankind.
Let them sacrifice thank offerings
and tell of his works with songs of joy.*

—Psalm 107:17–22 (NIV)

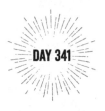

CHOOSE TO BELIEVE THE BEST ABOUT PEOPLE

Don't jump to conclusions. Don't assume the worst. Don't be judgmental and quick to write people off. Fight your cynical, pessimistic urges, which keep you in a state of suspicion and paranoia.

Believing the best about people isn't clueless naiveté. It's choosing to believe a reasonable non-nefarious explanation of someone's motives in the absence of evidence when you are tempted to suspect otherwise.

Do unto others as you would have them do unto you. People mean well, and most folks are doing the best they can. Give them the benefit of the doubt. Choose to believe the best about people.

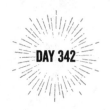

FUTURE LIFE MATH

All of your decisions add up over time.

They can add up to good results or not-so-good results.

Your life today is the sum total of all the decisions you've made in the past.

Your decisions—yes, mostly your decisions—got you here.

And your future life will be created by the decisions you make going forward, starting now.

Your future is not preprogrammed. You are not a victim of fate.

Your destiny is determined by you.

Your daily choices matter.

You can make better decisions and get better results.

Choose to take care of yourself. Choose to give your body an abundance of nutrition. Choose to exercise. Choose to give your worries and fears to God and trust Him with your future. Choose to love your enemies and forgive those who hurt you.

Make good choices today!

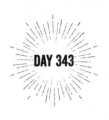

DAY 343

BE STRONG AND COURAGEOUS, DO NOT BE AFRAID OR TREMBLE AT THEM, FOR THE LORD YOUR GOD IS THE ONE WHO GOES WITH YOU. HE WILL NOT FAIL YOU OR FORSAKE YOU.

—DEUTERONOMY 31:6 (NASB)

HONOR YOUR PARENTS

*Honor your father and mother. Then you will live a long,
full life in the land the Lord your God is giving you.*

—Exodus 19:12 (NLT)

This is one of the Ten Commandments, so it's safe to say it's
pretty important. And there is a promise attached to this
command: a long, full life.

Notice that this command is not conditional. It doesn't
say "honor your father and mother if they are worthy" or
"honor your father and mother when you are together" or
"honor your father and mother as long as they are alive." It
just says honor your father and mother. Period.

The way you live your life can bring honor or shame on
your parents. And this commandment implies that if you
don't honor your parents, you may not live a long, full life.
So let's not take any chances.

If you have dishonored your parents in the past through
your words or actions, repent, apologize if applicable, make
changes, and make a decision to honor them going forward.
Love them, serve them, speak kind words to them and about
them, and do not expose their flaws and failures. And let
your life story be one that they are proud to tell.

Honor your parents. Then you will live a long, full life
in the land the Lord your God is giving you.

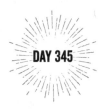

SURRENDER

Some battles aren't worth fighting. Some battles end up hurting you more than anyone else, even if you win. They waste your time, energy, and money. They exhaust you mentally, emotionally, and spiritually.

There's a time to fight and there's a time to surrender, and sometimes surrendering is the wisest thing you can do.

Surrender your pride, surrender your ego, surrender your need to be right, surrender your grudges, surrender your guilt, surrender your shame, surrender your resentment, and surrender your sin.

Surrender to your new life. Surrender to change and to growth.

Surrender is not an act of weakness. It is an act of strength and trust.

Surrender your life to your Heavenly Father, who loves you with an unconditional everlasting love, and trust that He will lead you on the path of healing.

Today's Challenge: *Ask yourself:* In which areas of my life do I need to stand firm and fight and in which areas do I need to surrender?

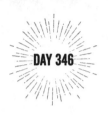

IF WE COULD READ THE SECRET HISTORY OF OUR ENEMIES, WE SHOULD FIND IN EACH MAN'S LIFE SORROW AND SUFFERING ENOUGH TO DISARM ALL HOSTILITY.

—HENRY WADSWORTH LONGFELLOW

Remember this about your enemies. Those who inflict pain on others are also suffering. God loves them as much as He loves you.

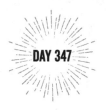

WALK LIKE AN EGYPTIAN . . . EXILE

We walk by faith, not by sight.

—2 Corinthians 5:7

Walking by sight is easy. It's easy when your eyes are open, and you can see a clear path to your destination. It's easy when you have a map and a handbook. It's easy when you can see the risks, obstacles, and dangerous terrain up ahead and avoid them.

But often in life, you find yourself facing obstacles you didn't expect. It's like the lights go out and you're stumbling around in the dark. You have no idea what's ahead of you. You can't even see the next step.

Or what you *can* see, the mountains you have to cross, the giants you have to face and fight, prevents you from moving forward into your destiny, your Promised Land.

Walking by faith is embracing the difficult journey, stepping out into the unknown, into scary, uncharted territory, believing that God will supply all of your needs: that He will clear a path for you, that He will make a way where there is no way, that He will direct your steps and carry you when you feel like you can't take another one, and that He will never leave you or forsake you. We walk by faith, not by sight!

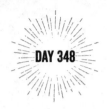

CHOOSE TODAY

Yesterday is over. It's in the past. You can't change it. So let it go.

Don't live in a state of regret, dwelling on your mistakes and continually beating yourself up.

Tomorrow is out of your reach and out of your control.

You can plan for tomorrow, but don't worry about what might happen.

The only thing you have control over are the choices you make right now in this moment. *Today.*

Today's choices produce tomorrow's results.

Your choices matter. So, it makes sense to make good choices today.

Choose to live. Choose to be joyful. Choose to be thankful. Choose to be positive. Choose to forgive. Choose to love others. And choose to love yourself with healthy choices.

Each day you have the opportunity to sow seeds of health or disease. Sow good seeds. The harvest is coming!

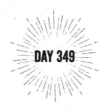

#TURTLEPOWER

*Behold the turtle. He only makes progress
when he sticks his neck out.*

—OFTEN ATTRIBUTED TO JAMES BRYANT CONANT

Sticking your neck out is risky, but you have to stick your neck out and get going. And even though some days may feel like your progress is turtle-slow, remember . . .

Slow and steady wins the race.
—Aesop

So be persistent like a turtle and keep moving forward a little bit more every day. Also be glad you aren't actually a turtle because . . .

All the thoughts of a turtle are turtles.
—Ralph Waldo Emerson

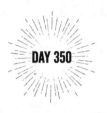

STOP BEING OFFENDED

One of the greatest privileges we have in the United States, and many other countries, is free speech. Free speech means you have the legal right to say anything you want as long as you aren't threatening to physically harm someone else. It means you have the freedom to voice your opinion and your beliefs. It also means other people have the freedom to voice their opinions and beliefs that you don't like. These days, it seems like everyone is offended by everything. People are looking for things to get offended about. They're getting offended by proxy, on behalf of other people who aren't even offended.

In the last 10 years, as a public figure I've been criticized and attacked in painful and offensive ways more times than I can count. It used to hurt my feelings. But I don't get offended anymore because I realized that being offended is a choice, and living in a perpetual state of offense and outrage is a formula for lasting unhappiness and a miserable existence.

Here's the truth: Some people are mean. And mean people say offensive things because they want your attention and they want to offend you. And if you get offended, they win. You are giving them power and control over your mental and emotional state. But if you choose not to be offended, you win.

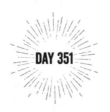

PESSIMISM MAKES YOUR LIFE WORSE

If you are a pessimist in the sense that when bad things happen you think they are going to last forever and undermine everything you do, then you are about eight times as likely to get depressed, you are less likely to succeed at work, your personal relationships are more likely to break up, and you are likely to have a shorter and more illness-filled life.

—Martin E. P. Seligman, Ph.D.

Pessimism is simply an unhealthy pattern of thought and self-talk. It's a bad habit that you can break and replace with optimism. In order to do this, you must dispute the catastrophic thinking and false accusations that you make against yourself. That you can't . . . that you aren't good enough . . . that you will always be [insert something negative] . . . that bad things always happen to you . . . that no one loves you . . . that you will never get well. Reject those thoughts.

Believe that bad things that happen to you, like cancer, are temporary, not permanent.

Believe that you have control over your life, your health, and your future. And believe that good things are coming!

DAY 352

THE FEAR OF THE LORD PROLONGS LIFE, BUT THE YEARS OF THE WICKED ARE CUT SHORT.

—PROVERBS 10:27 (HCSB)

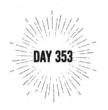

PROMISE YOURSELF

*To be so strong that nothing can disturb your peace of mind.
To forget the mistakes of the past and press on to
the greater achievements of the future.
To give so much time to the improvement of yourself
that you have no time to criticize others.
To be too large for worry, too noble for anger, too strong
for fear, and too happy to permit the presence of trouble.*

—Christian D. Larson, *The Optimist Creed*

DAY 354

Never attribute to malice that which is adequately explained by stupidity.

—ROBERT J. HANLON

Everybody makes mistakes, and sometimes those mistakes cause problems or harm. But don't jump to the conclusion that the harm was intentional. Rather, choose to believe that it was an honest (or maybe stupid) mistake. Hey, we all make 'em.

The humorous maxim quoted above, known as Hanlon's Razor, is useful when you find yourself confused about another person's actions or motives. It will prevent your imagination from running wild with conspiracy theories, thereby leading you to assume the worst, get angry, overreact, stir up a bunch of drama, and make a scene in front of your family, friends, coworkers, strangers, or all those people scrutinizing your every move on social media.

Choose to believe the best about people, rather than assuming the worst.

Having said that, chronic problem-causers may require closer scrutiny. Some people are so overwhelmingly inconsiderate and selfish by nature that they constantly cause stress, anxiety, and problems for everyone around them. Regardless of the explanation (malice or stupidity), for your own sanity and peace of mind, I recommend you distance yourself from people like this.

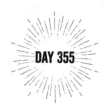

DAY 355

*No power in society, no hardship in your condition,
can depress you, keep you down, in knowledge, power,
virtue, influence, but by your own consent.*

—WILLIAM ELLERY CHANNING

Ignorant, powerless, immoral, and ineffectual . . . These
are not the qualities of the person you were created to be.
Do not consent! You were created for great things. And you
have the resources of heaven at your disposal. Rise up and
take back your power!

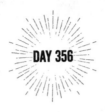

THE DAY I GOT RICH . . .

In 2015, I visited an orphanage in Cambodia founded by my friend Sean Ngu. These kids were not typical orphans. Their parents had died of AIDS and all the kids were HIV positive. Their extended families had refused to adopt them out of fear of the disease.

We spent the afternoon playing with the kids, and we gave them treats and snacks, hugged them, and loved on them. They were smiling, laughing, and running around, just like kids do. We walked through the building and I saw their bunk beds and their little bits of clothing and the gravity of their life hit me. These children had truly had nothing—no parents, no belongings—and they had HIV/AIDS.

My heart broke for these kids, and I realized how rich I was just to grow up in a home with parents, clothing, toys, and health. I felt so ashamed for ever complaining about anything.

So when things aren't going your way, when you're having a bad day, or when you're feeling envious of others or down on yourself, remember that there are people in the world with nothing. Count your blessings and remind yourself how rich you are. This will transform your perspective. You will have so much gratitude in your heart when you focus on the abundance of good things you have in your life.

DAY 357

Practical life advice from the Apostle Paul to the church in Thessalonica:

> *We urge you, brethren, admonish the unruly, encourage the fainthearted, help the weak, be patient with everyone.*
>
> *See that no one repays another with evil for evil, but always seek after that which is good for one another and for all people.*
>
> *Rejoice always; pray without ceasing; in everything give thanks; for this is God's will for you in Christ Jesus.*
> —1 Thessalonians 5:14–18 (NASB)

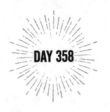

DAY 358

FILE NOT FOUND . . .

If you don't have clarity . . . if you are unsure about your next steps . . . if you feel confused . . . if you don't understand your options . . . if you can't make up your mind about what to do . . .

You don't have enough information.

And if you don't have enough information, you cannot make a wise decision.

Tell yourself, tell your family, tell your doctors, "I need more information."

And then take the time to gather it.

Ask more questions. Get more opinions. Do more research. Read articles and books. Talk to more doctors and survivors. And pray for guidance. Wisdom and clarity will come. And then you can make an informed decision and take your next steps with confidence.

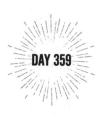

DAY 359

THE HORSE IS PREPARED FOR THE DAY OF BATTLE, BUT VICTORY BELONGS TO THE LORD.

—PROVERBS 21:31 (NASB)

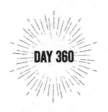

BE GENEROUS

Give, and it will be given to you. A good measure, pressed down, shaken together and running over, will be poured into your lap. For with the measure you use, it will be measured to you.

—Jesus
—Luke 6:38 (NIV)

You reap what you sow. What goes around comes around. Give generously and you will receive generously. It truly is better to give than to receive. And the beautiful thing about giving is that it sets you up to receive more! And you can't outgive God!

Today I want to challenge you to be generous. Be more generous than you ever have been before. Not just on holidays or birthdays. Look for ways to bless people that come into your life. Give to everyone who asks of you. Become the most generous person you know.

Give love and affection, give your time, give your attention, give money, give food or clothing, give away things you don't need.

Here's an easy thing: Keep extra cash in your wallet specifically to give to those in need when the opportunity arises. Jesus also said when you give, do it secretly. Your Heavenly Father sees it and will reward you (Matthew 6:3–4)!

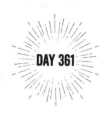

"HE [JESUS] HIMSELF BORE OUR SINS" IN HIS BODY ON THE CROSS, SO THAT WE MIGHT DIE TO SINS AND LIVE FOR RIGHTEOUSNESS; "BY HIS WOUNDS YOU HAVE BEEN HEALED."

—1 PETER 2:24 (NIV)

Thank you, Jesus, that you bore my sin and sickness on the cross and that by your stripes I am healed!

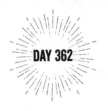

POSITIVELY CHANGE YOUR BRAIN AND BODY

A study of over 4,000 people with an average age of 72 found that those with a positive attitude about aging were 50 percent less likely to develop dementia—even if they carried the gene most linked to dementia. But the people who faced aging with pessimism and fear were more likely to suffer from dementia.

Another study found that negative thinkers who ruminated on the past, worried about the future, and focused on their problems had increased deposits of tau and beta amyloid in their brains, two proteins linked to higher rates of cognitive decline such as Alzheimer's and dementia.[41]

Stress is a root cause of chronic disease. Negative thoughts and emotions produce harmful chemical reactions that promote inflammation throughout your body, suppress your immune system, and damage your brain. Negative thoughts can outweigh your healthy habits and undermine your healing.

Here's how to retrain your brain: Release your past. Practice gratitude. Meditate and pray. Catch those negative thoughts and reject them. Give your worries and fears to God. Choose to think positively and visualize your Best Possible Self healthy and thriving in the future.[42] Jesus said it best: "Don't worry about tomorrow, for today has enough trouble of its own" (Matthew 6:34).

---

41 Marchant et al., "Repetitive Negative Thinking Is Associated with Amyloid, Tau, and Cognitive Decline," *Alzheimers & Dementia* 16, no. 7 (July 2020): 1054–1064.
42 J. M. Malouff and N. S. Schutte, "Can Psychological Interventions Increase Optimism? A Meta-Analysis," *The Journal of Positive Psychology* 12, no. 6 (2017): 594–604.

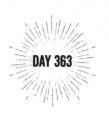

DAY 363

TOUGH TIMES NEVER LAST, BUT TOUGH PEOPLE DO!

—ROBERT H. SCHULLER

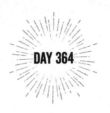

SWIM SIDEWAYS

Life is like the ocean. There are multiple currents moving in different directions. Some currents take you exactly where you want to go. Some take you to surprising, wonderful new places. Some take you in circles. Some take you way off course. And some currents can be life threatening.

If you are swimming in the ocean and you get caught in a riptide, it will quickly pull you away from the shore. A riptide is a current so powerful that you cannot swim against it. You cannot fight it. Doing so will exhaust you. And eventually you drown. The way to survive a riptide is to swim sideways until you get out of the current. Then you can swim back to shore.

Some currents in life are too strong to swim against. They are too powerful to overcome directly. Consider your options . . .

You can surrender and let the current take you out to sea. You can swim against it with all of your might, and maybe, miraculously, you will prevail. Or you can outsmart it by getting out of the current.

You can always swim sideways.

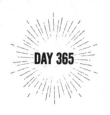

DAY 365

PEACE I LEAVE WITH YOU; MY PEACE I GIVE TO YOU; NOT AS THE WORLD GIVES DO I GIVE TO YOU. DO NOT LET YOUR HEART BE TROUBLED, NOR LET IT BE FEARFUL.

—JESUS
—JOHN 14:27 (NASB)

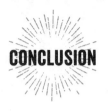

CONCLUSION

I love it when a plan comes together.
—Colonel John "Hannibal" Smith, *The A-Team*

Congratulations! You made it to the end of *Beat Cancer Daily*! Did you actually read and focus on one page per day, or did you blaze through it? Tag me **@chrisbeatcancer #beatcancerdaily** on social media and let me know.

Either way, I hope these pages have inspired you to radically change your life.

And now that you are at the end of the book, I have a suggestion for you . . .

I think you should you start over on Day 1!

This book will keep encouraging and inspiring you over and over again. And it will be even better the second time. I promise!

My prayer for you is from Numbers 6:24–26 (NIV):

The Lord bless you and keep you; the Lord make His face shine on you and be gracious to you; the Lord turn his face toward you and give you peace.

Love,
Chris

ACKNOWLEDGMENTS

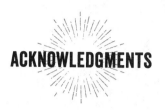

It should be noted for future readers that the majority of this book was written in the midst of the COVID-19 pandemic, a time of unprecedented levels fear and uncertainty—unprecedented in my 43 years of life, anyway. School was canceled, movie theaters closed, events were canceled, travel stopped. Millions of people around the globe were unable to work, and we were under quarantine or were sheltering at home for months. Social distancing and mask wearing in public became the norm. In some ways the world got a taste of what everyday life is like for cancer patients. When your life gets turned upside down, you lose all sense of normalcy, and you become acutely aware of the impending threat of debilitating illness and death, you realize what really matters and how much you had taken for granted. And you cherish those things. Storms come and go in life. And like all storms, this too shall pass. The person who builds their house on a solid foundation can weather every storm of life (Matthew 7:24–27).

Thank you to my incredible wife and my dream girl, Micah, and to my two beautiful daughters, Marin and Mackenzie. I love you all with all of my heart, more than the whole wide world.

Thank you to Dr. Leigh Erin Connealy, Dr. Kristi Funk, Theo and Kim Hanson, Kevin and Cortney Campbell, Suzy Griswold, Julie Johnson, Ivelisse Page, and Paula Black for your inspired contributions to this volume!

Thank you to everyone at Hay House who helped bring this book to life. Thank you to Reid Tracy and Patty Gift for believing in me and my message. Thank you to my editor

Lisa Cheng for your guidance and support. Thank you to Tricia Breidenthal for your patience with me and my countless cover and interior design iterations.

And finally, thank you to my fellow unwitting members of the Cancer Club. You inspire me every day with your determination and courage. May all of your days be filled with peace, love, and joy.

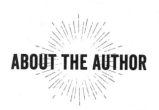

ABOUT THE AUTHOR

Chris Wark is the best-selling author of *Chris Beat Cancer: A Comprehensive Plan for Healing Naturally*. He is a patient advocate, a speaker, and a health coach. Chris was diagnosed with stage III colon cancer in 2003 at 26 years old. He had surgery, but instead of chemotherapy, he used nutrition and natural therapies to heal himself. Chris has made many appearances on radio and television and was featured in the award-winning documentary film *The C Word*. Chris inspires countless people to take control of their health and reverse disease with a radical transformation of diet and lifestyle. You can visit him online at **www.chrisbeatcancer.com**.

Also by Chris Wark

Chris Beat Cancer

The above is available at your local bookstore,
or may be ordered by visiting:

Hay House USA: www.hayhouse.com®
Hay House Australia: www.hayhouse.com.au
Hay House UK: www.hayhouse.co.uk
Hay House India: www.hayhouse.co.in

Hay House Titles of Related Interest

YOU CAN HEAL YOUR LIFE, the movie,
starring Louise Hay & Friends
(available as an online streaming video)
www.hayhouse.com/louise-movie

THE SHIFT, the movie,
starring Dr. Wayne W. Dyer
(available as an online streaming video)
www.hayhouse.com/the-shift-movie

*CANCER-FREE WITH FOOD: A Step-by-Step Plan with
100+ Recipes to Fight Disease, Nourish Your Body & Restore
Your Health*, by Liana Werner-Gray

*CRAZY SEXY JUICE: 100+ Simple Juice, Smoothie & Nut
Milk Recipes to Supercharge Your Health,* by Kris Carr

All of the above are available at your local bookstore,
or may be ordered by contacting Hay House (see next page).

We hope you enjoyed this Hay House book. If you'd like to receive our online catalog featuring additional information on Hay House books and products, or if you'd like to find out more about the Hay Foundation, please contact:

Hay House LLC, P.O. Box 5100, Carlsbad, CA 92018-5100
(760) 431-7695 or (800) 654-5126
www.hayhouse.com® • www.hayfoundation.org

———

Published in Australia by:
Hay House Australia Publishing Pty Ltd
18/36 Ralph St., Alexandria NSW 2015
Phone: +61 (02) 9669 4299
www.hayhouse.com.au

Published in the United Kingdom by:
Hay House UK Ltd
The Sixth Floor, Watson House,
54 Baker Street, London W1U 7BU
Phone: +44 (0) 203 927 7290
www.hayhouse.co.uk

Published in India by:
Hay House Publishers (India) Pvt Ltd
Muskaan Complex, Plot No. 3,
B-2, Vasant Kunj, New Delhi 110 070
Phone: +91 11 41761620
www.hayhouse.co.in

———

Let Your Soul Grow

Experience life-changing transformation—one video at a time—with guidance from the world's leading experts.

www.healyourlifeplus.com

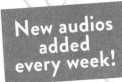